COLOR ME MENOPAUSAL

Quarto.com • WalterFoster.com

© 2025 Quarto Publishing Group USA Inc.
Illustrations © 2025 Veronica Carratello

Written by Shirley Șerban

First Published in 2025 by Walter Foster Publishing,
an imprint of The Quarto Group,
100 Cummings Center, Suite 265-D, Beverly, MA 01915, USA.
T (978) 282-9590 F (978) 283-2742

The information in this book is not intended to replace the medical advice of a qualified physician. Consult with your doctor before using the information in this or any health-related publication.

Walter Foster Publishing titles are also available at discount for retail, wholesale, promotional, and bulk purchase. For details, contact the Special Sales Manager by email at specialsales@quarto.com or by mail at The Quarto Group, Attn: Special Sales Manager, 100 Cummings Center, Suite 265-D, Beverly, MA 01915, USA.

29 28 27 26 25   1 2 3 4 5

ISBN: 978-0-7603-9248-5

Design and Page Layout: Mattie Wells Design LLC

Printed in China

COLOR ME MENOPAUSAL

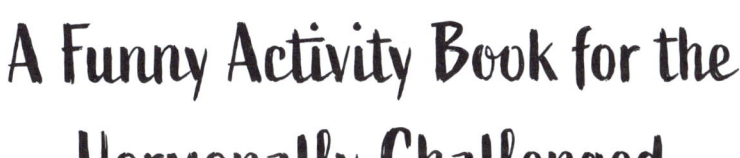

A Funny Activity Book for the Hormonally Challenged

Shirley Șerban

Illustrated by Veronica Carratello

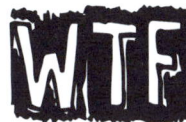

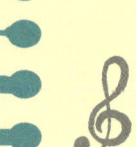

Is this my new life?

Irritability?

Shutting down inside

I can't sleep and am so itchy

Got sweaty thighs

This is my demise, you see...

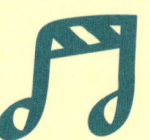

MENOPAUSE RHAPSODY

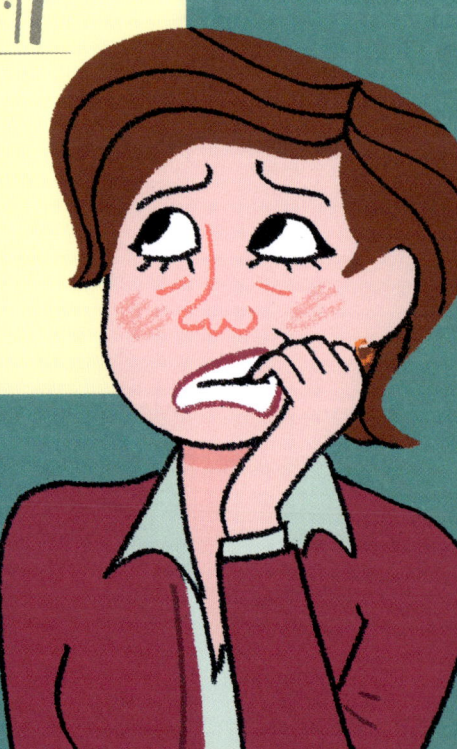

INTRODUCTION

Hi! I'm Shirley, and I'm guessing I might be a bit like you—going from a complete novice in all things menopause to finding myself in the hot, sweaty mess of riding this new hormonal roller coaster!

I wrote the lyrics on the previous page a couple of years ago for fun, as part of a parody to "Bohemian Rhapsody" by Queen. My "Menopause Rhapsody" seemed to strike a chord worldwide and thrust me into the spotlight as some kind of menopause expert. To overcome my imposter syndrome, I dug deeper, and found that I was in the midst of perimenopause without even realizing it!

Welcome to menopause, with all its ups and downs. It feels a tad unfair, doesn't it? We've endured decades of cramps, periods, PMS, bloating—the whole shebang— only to be greeted by this! Our reproductive organs' swan song is more like a tone-deaf warble: hot flashes, night sweats, and weight gain, oh my!

The reality is that perimenopause (because that's really when the hard work happens) is a challenging time, so why not have a good laugh and maybe a good cry about it? This book is for you, because, let's be honest, the media and your run-of-the-mill doctor's office won't spill the menopausal tea. (Did you know most women just want to normalize what's happening to them?)

With this book, I hope you'll kick back, relax, maybe color outside the lines, quiz yourself, and chuckle at the realization that your body is doing what bodies do. You're not alone; there are legions of kindred spirits muttering under their breath about enduring sleepless nights, sprouting new chin hairs, and shedding tears over nothing. So, fire off a text to your BFF, share your "Aha!" moment, or spill the beans about that laugh-until-you-pee incident. Heck, gift a copy to your friend and plan your very own menopause party. We've got this!

YOU AND YOUR MENOPAUSE

Since this book is all about you and your changing parts, the good, the bad, and the itchy, tell us all about it! Fill in the blanks.

My name is _____.

I am _____ years old. I was _____ when I first started my period.

I started getting irregular periods when I was _____.

This means I've had about _____ years of having regular periods.
(subtract your age of starting your period from your age of starting irregular periods)

That's about _____ periods!
(multiply the last answer by 12)

My regular periods would normally last for _____ days.

This means, I've been surfing the crimson wave for about _____ days!
(multiply the above answer by the previous answer)

Other things I had to deal with on a monthly basis with my regular periods were:
(Select all that applied to you)

o Cramps   o Acne   o Migraines   o Other:
o PMS   o Sore joints   o Mood Swings   _____
o Bloating   o Headaches   o NEED for
                                      comfort food

So now I'm in perimenopause / menopause.
(circle which best applies)

But HELLO, look at my stats! I've been dealing with all those symptoms (and doing it with style, I might add) for so long! Bring out the party hats and streamers and give my hoo-ha a break. I welcome this freeing stage of my life!

WHAT WILL MY DAY LOOK LIKE?

The path you choose will determine your future . . . I'm no fortune teller, but start at the center, and this maze will predict your day. (Hint: There's more than one answer!)

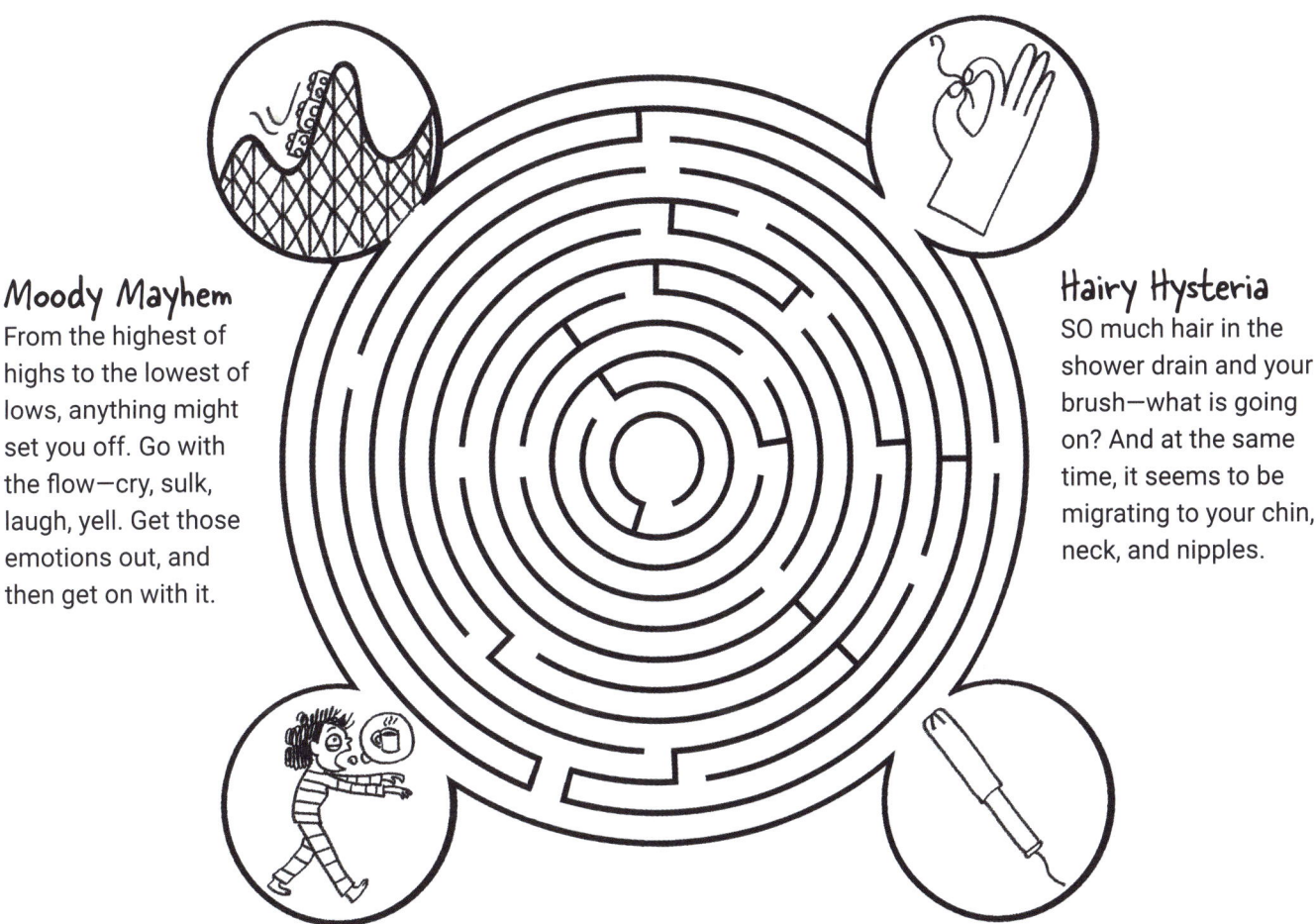

Moody Mayhem
From the highest of highs to the lowest of lows, anything might set you off. Go with the flow—cry, sulk, laugh, yell. Get those emotions out, and then get on with it.

Hairy Hysteria
SO much hair in the shower drain and your brush—what is going on? And at the same time, it seems to be migrating to your chin, neck, and nipples.

Sleepy Zombie You've been up half the night with sweats, needing to pee, or just stuck on a 3 a.m. thought that has made you anxious. No wonder you're now standing at the open fridge, wondering what on earth you're doing. Go back to bed!

Surprise! It's back! You were getting excited about your periods disappearing, but one decides to come and visit today, right when you didn't need it. Carry extra supplies, and prepare for some PMS and cramping.

Answer on page 92.

CELEBRITIES—THEY'RE JUST LIKE US

If you were born with a female reproductive system and you make it to middle age, there's no escaping menopause, even if you're famous! Read the following quotes and try matching them to the celeb who said each one.

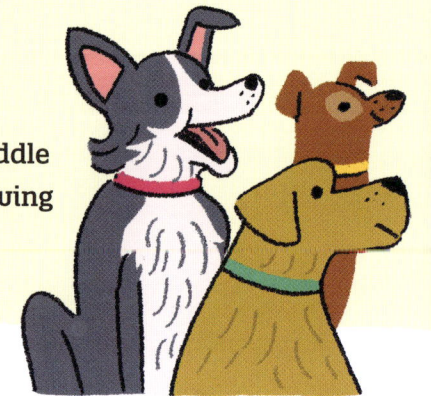

CELEBRITIES:

Shania Twain

Oprah Winfrey

Michelle Yeoh

Michelle Obama

Emma Thompson

Viola Davis

Joan Rivers

Drew Barrymore

Halle Berry

Angelina Jolie

Salma Hayek

CELEBRITY QUOTES:

1. "A study says owning a dog makes you 10 years younger. My first thought was to rescue two more, but I don't want to go through menopause again."

   _____

2. "We're all in menopause with stretchy [waist] bands and our athleisure wear on, and you look up and you can't fit the outfits you had last year."

   _____

3. "It's such a cold night. You know, it's the first time I've been actively grateful for the menopause."

   _____

4. "I will not be able to have any more children, and I expect some physical changes. But I feel at ease with whatever will come, not because I am strong but because this is a part of life. It is nothing to be feared."

   _____

5. "Menopause taught me to quickly say, 'You know, it may only get worse. So just love yourself now.'"

   _____

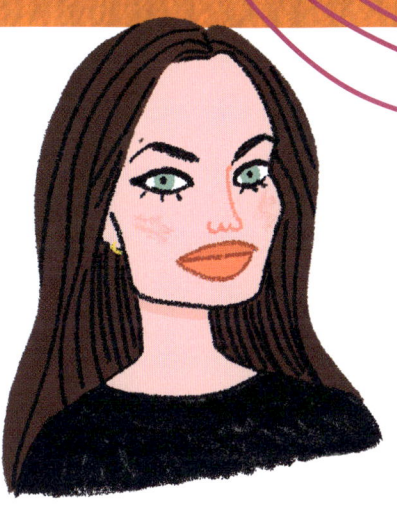

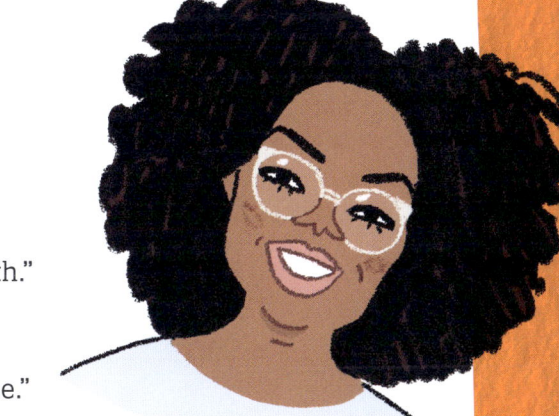

6. "When you talk about menopause, men just die . . . a slow death."

_____

7. "Ladies, don't let anybody tell you you are ever past your prime."

_____

8. "There's no expiration dates for women. That has to go. Because you can kick ass at any age. You can hold your own at any age, you can dream at any age, you can be romantic at age."

_____

9. "So many women I've talked to see menopause as a blessing. I've discovered that this is your moment to reinvent yourself after years of focusing on the needs of everyone else."

_____

10. "I'm smack dab in the middle of menopause, and I am challenging everything I thought I knew about menopause, like, 'your life is over. You are disposable. Society no longer has a place for you. That's not true. I'm my best self now that I reached 56 years old. I have the most to offer."

_____

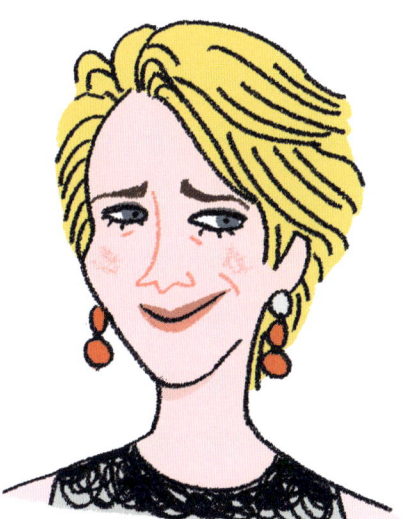

11. "One doctor also just told me, like, this could last, on the worst-case scenario, 10 years. And I was like, 'I will never make it 10 years like this."

_____

Answers on page 92.

MENOPAUSE-O-METER TEST

Am I menopausal? Wonder no more—we have designed a foolproof test. Check all the statements that are true for you and add up how many you selected at the end to find out where you are on the menopause-o-meter!

☐ I have a mental map of all the toilets at the mall.

☐ I'm either getting up to pee or to turn down the A/C every night.

☐ I just teared up watching a cute kitten video . . . so fluffy! So sweet!

☐ I had a period a few months ago, but no sign of it yet and no clue when or if it will come again.

☐ Tweezers are my new must-have accessory and I'm sure magnifying mirrors are the devil's work.

☐ I suddenly find the Hulk and Jekyll and Hyde super relatable—they're just misunderstood and trying their best.

☐ I'm not sure if I watched the latest "it" TV show—I have to ask my partner if I fell asleep again or not.

☐ Somehow all my pants shrank in the wash.

☐ Who needs to travel? I experience the tropics regularly without having to get on a plane.

☐ I forgot what this test was about—what are we doing here?

Total:_____

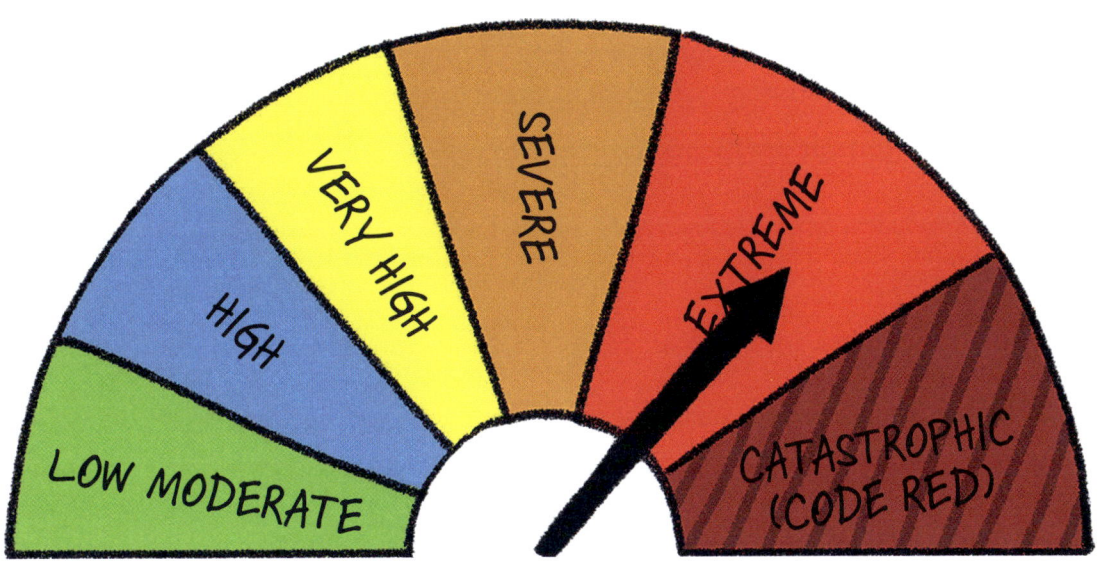

MENOPAUSE-O-METER

HOW MANY DID YOU SELECT?

0: Low–Moderate
You're either one of those hideously lucky things that breezes through life without a care in the world, or you're too young or have too many Y chromosomes for this book.

1–2: High
Karen Carpenter sang, "We've Only Just Begun." Looks like you're getting a couple of hints of perimenopause, and you're probably wondering what the fuss is all about. Enjoy these early days and buckle up!

3–4: Very High
Few may know you have perimenopausal symptoms, but you sure do. Oh, yes, and when you see someone else uncomfortable in a similar way, you give them a knowing nod or smile.

5–7: Severe
We hope the people you love get it. And if they're not, explain this to them! You've got this! So much is tough, but you are tougher.

8–9: Extreme
If menopause were an Olympic sport, you'd be a multi-athlete. Few realize how hard this is for you, and you plod on through regardless. Legend.

10: Catastrophic (Code Red)
Raging, raving, menopausal maniac! Hats off to you, sister—you are in the furnace now, but it'll all be over soon. Almost definitely less than fourteen years to go!

MENOPAUSE REGISTRY

Forget the Bridal Registry! Here are the things to add to your Menopause Registry.

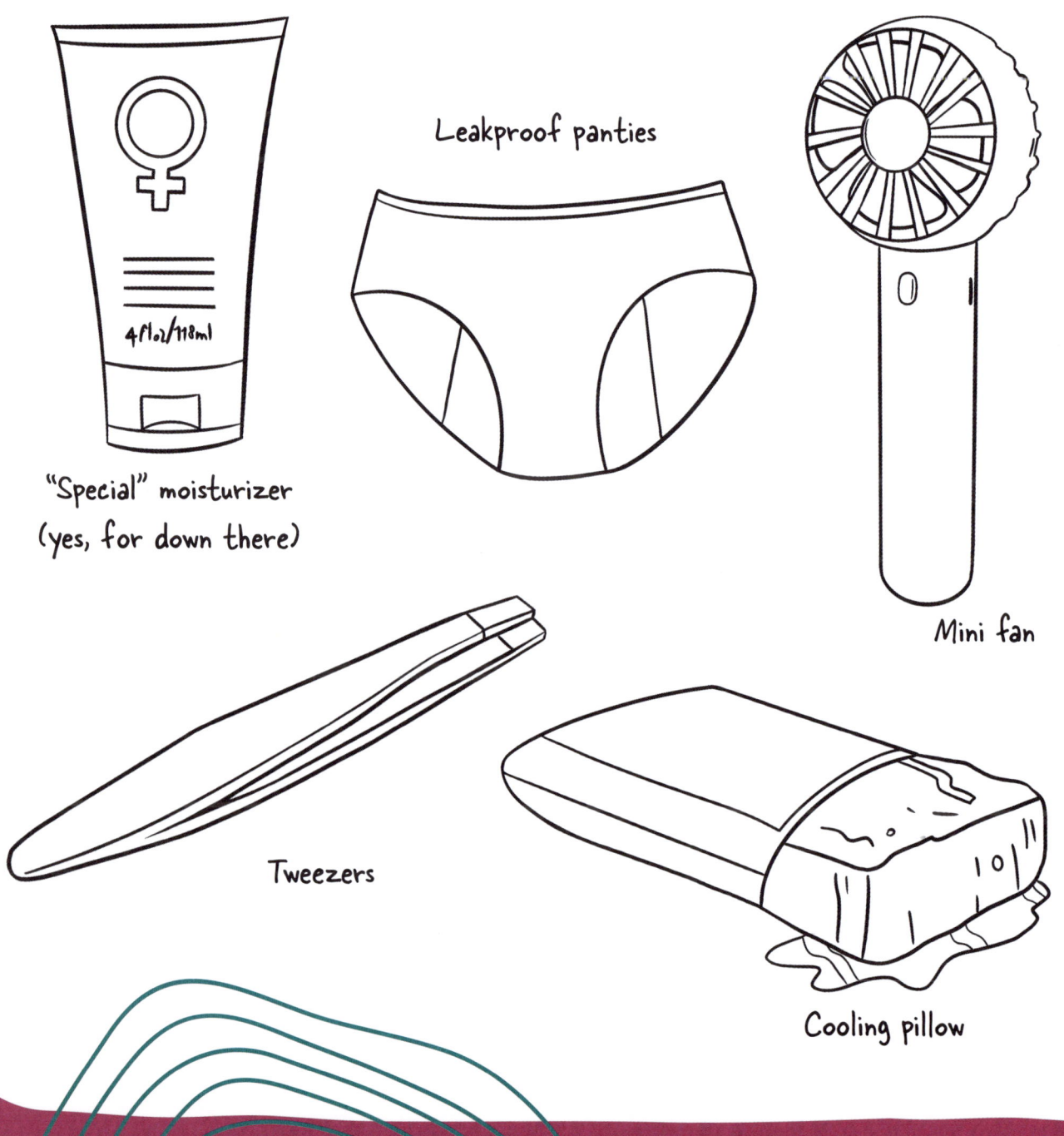

"Special" moisturizer
(yes, for down there)

Leakproof panties

Mini fan

Tweezers

Cooling pillow

4 fl oz/118ml

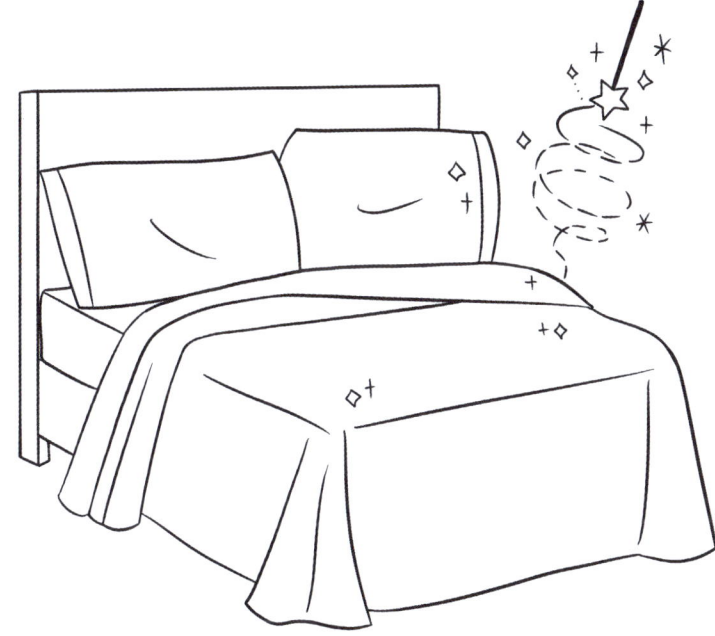

Magic, sweat-wicking sheets

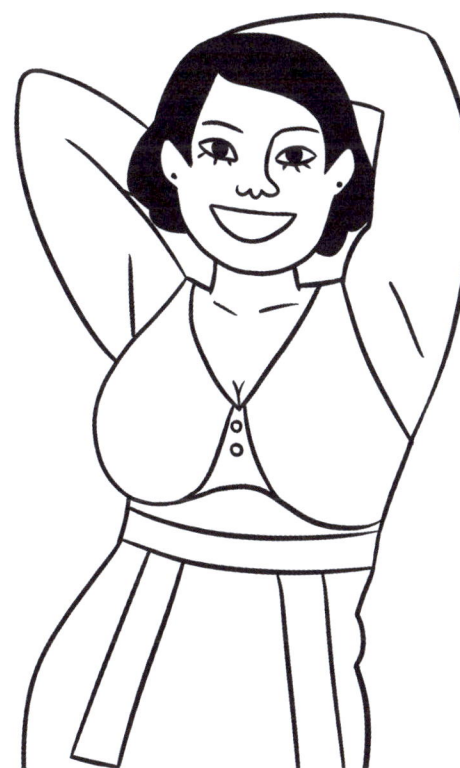

Shapewear

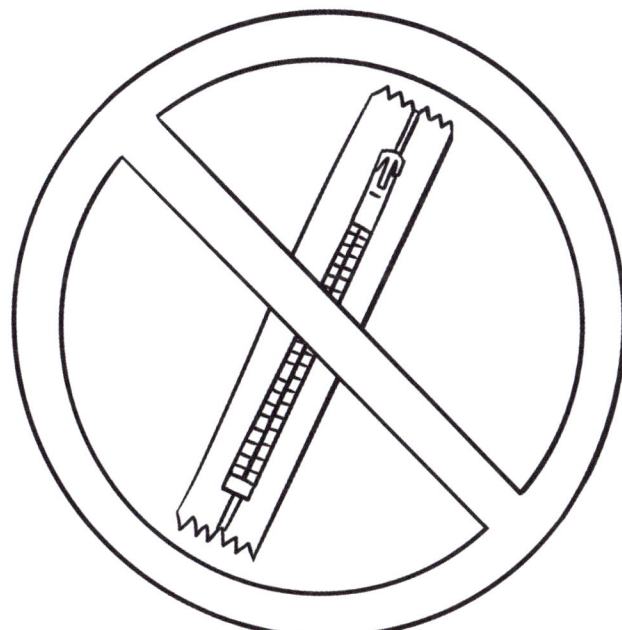

Clothing without zips, tight
buttons, or underwire

What else would you put on
your Menopause Registry?

WHAT WAS I THINKING?

Research suggests that up to two-thirds of those going through menopause experience the joys of brain fog. Where did I read that? I can't seem to remember . . . Unscramble the things I seem to lose track of most often, and use the letters they represent to solve the phrase at the end of the puzzle.

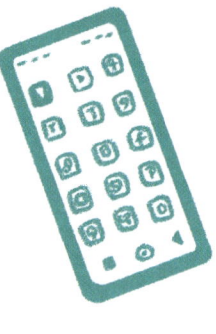

ESYK
☐☐☐☐
14 1

MPA
☐☐☐
44

ATDE
☐☐☐☐
18

MNSAE
☐☐☐☐☐
23 29

TSMNNITPPEAO
☐☐☐☐☐☐☐☐☐☐☐
20 21 35

DSORW
☐☐☐☐☐
19 32

NMTECAIODI
☐☐☐☐☐☐☐☐☐☐
37 31 25 7 45 41   46

VNNAASIREYR
☐☐☐☐☐☐☐☐☐☐☐
30 6

LTWAEL
☐☐☐☐☐☐
48   26 39

RDESSDA
☐☐☐☐☐☐☐
4   5

CRA
☐☐☐
33

HTDRSYBIA
☐☐☐☐☐☐☐☐☐
38 40 42   4/

RSEPU
☐☐☐☐☐
3

MEETOR
☐☐☐☐☐☐
34   10 36

YNURADL
☐☐☐☐☐☐☐
27   28   50

WOSSAPDR
☐☐☐☐☐☐☐☐
16   8

CSFAE
☐☐☐☐☐
17 49

NPE
☐☐☐
9

NHOEP
☐☐☐☐☐
2   24

SAELSGS
☐☐☐☐☐☐☐
12 15 43

ARTHS
☐☐☐☐☐
13 11 22

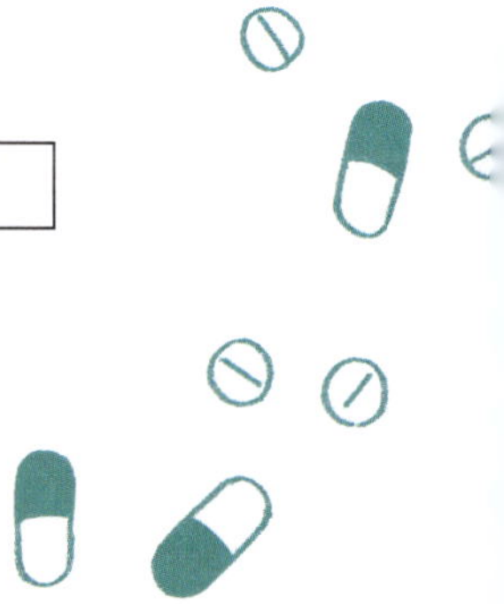

☐☐☐☐   ☐☐☐☐☐☐☐   ☐☐☐   ☐☐☐☐   ☐☐☐☐
1 2 3 4   5 6 7 8 9 10 11   12 13 14   15 16 17 18   19 20 21 22

☐☐.   ☐'☐☐   ☐☐☐☐☐   ☐☐☐☐☐☐☐☐
23 24   25 26 27   28 29 30 31 32   33 34 35 36 37 38 39 40

☐☐☐☐   ☐☐☐☐☐☐!
41 42 43 44   45 46 47 48 49 50

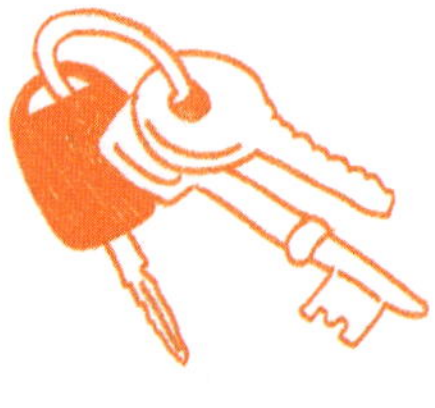

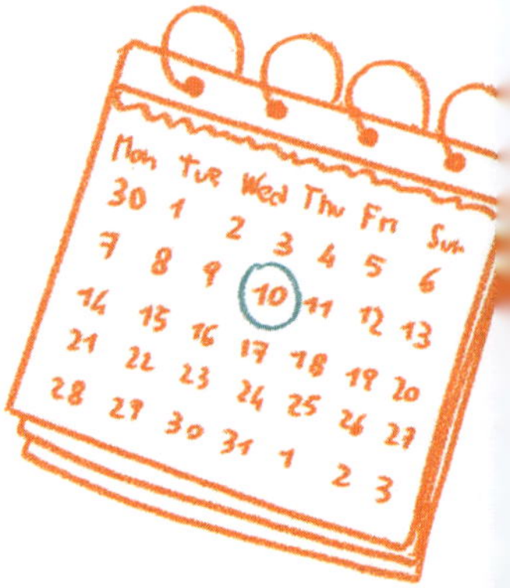

Answers on page 92.

DO YOU SPEAK BRAIN FART MENOSPEAK? I'M FLUENT

Have you ever been completely stumped at what something (or someone) is called? Embarrassing much? Estrogen impacts our brain function, and while it fluctuates during this stage of life, it means that even the simplest words can be just out of reach. Here are some things to say when you can't quite remember . . .

People's names when talking about them:

- Whatzisname
- You know who I mean, right?
- That one with a face
- That actor that was in that movie...

People's names when talking to someone:

- Just call them a pet name, like Sweetie, Dear, Honey, Sugar Pie, etc.
- Hey there...
- Hey, you!
- I want you to meet... (then pregnant pause waiting for them to say their name)

Place names:

- That, uh, that place down the road
- Ah, the name slips my mind...
- You know the one?
- The place where (describe in detail what happens there)

Things' names:

- Oh... you know... The ummm... thingy...
- That, uh, oh, what's it called again?

Now you try it! Translate these simple sentences into menospeak, where your brain has farted out the nouns! What might you say instead?

I want to go to the **grocery store** to buy some **soup**.

_____

I'm going to **Amy's wedding** in **Las Vegas**.

_____

(Partner or best friend's name)! Please come help me unload the **car**!

_____

Final bonus: Try ordering your favorite coffee or drink to go in Brain Fart Menospeak!

_____

NOT JUST SURVIVING, BUT THRIVING!

Did you know that the results of a 2019 survey of over six thousand "perimenopausers" found that this is a time of thriving, with many respondents caring more about their health; feeling happier, more confident, and physically strong; and with more disposable income and control in their careers?

Think about the things you're rocking and proud of at this stage in your life. Write your name on the trophy and draw or write these achievements in the spaces around it. Pity? No need, girl. You're killing it!

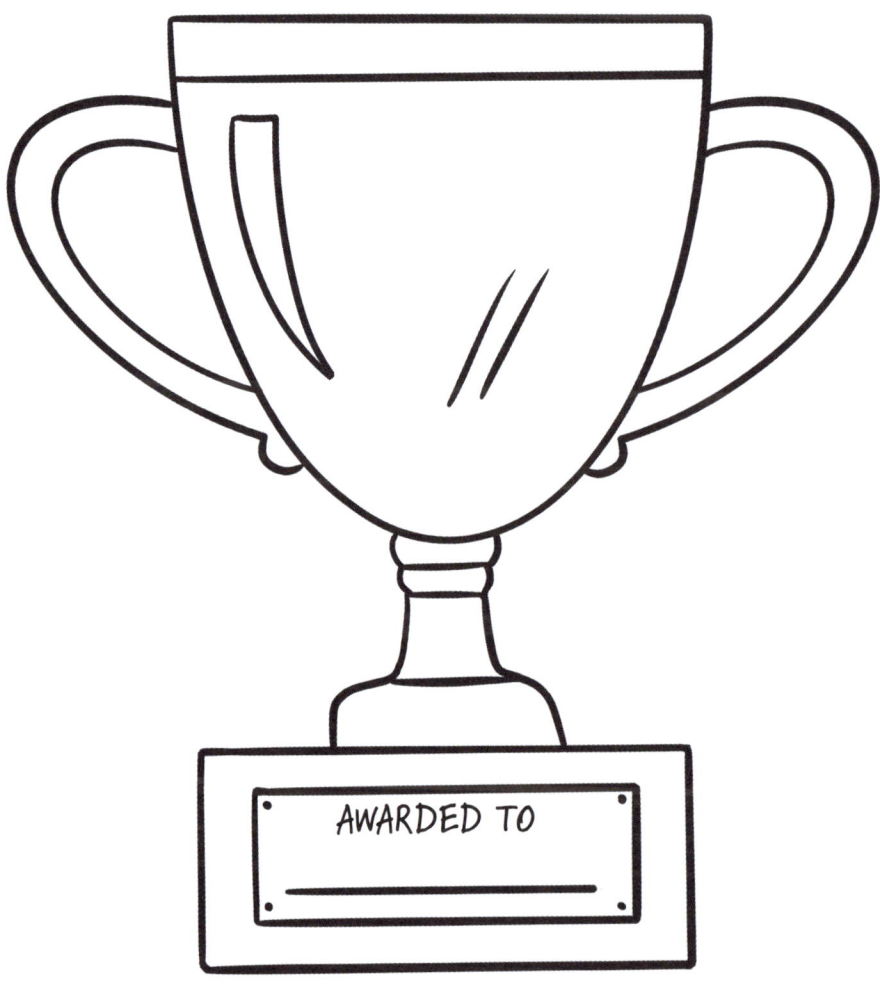

AWARDED TO

_____

FOR NOT LETTING THE DIFFICULTIES OF PERIMENOPAUSE
STOP THEM FROM ACHIEVING INCREDIBLE THINGS!

OH, PLEASE, PERIMENOPAUSE IS A BREEZE!

TIPS TO HIDE YOUR NEW REALITY FROM OTHERS

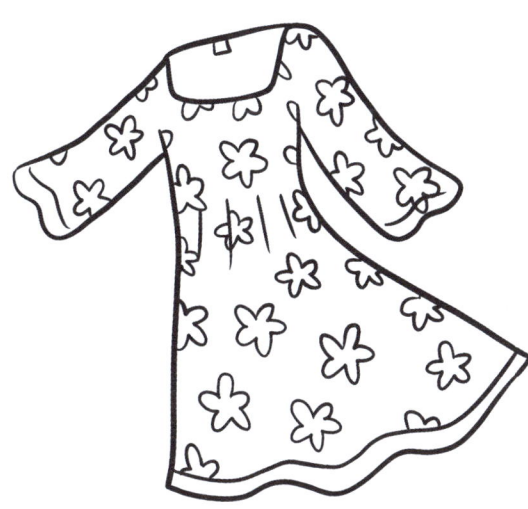

- Accidentally drop a tampon from your handbag, "Oops. That time of month! My bad."

- Bring back baggy, empire-waist dresses. Nobody will notice the changing tummy!

- Hang out outside hot yoga studios (people will presume you've taken a break, when you are really having a hot flash).

- Set your phone alarm to go off every few minutes. Each time it goes off, "answer" it and excuse yourself—important business to tend to. This gives you the opportunity to empty your bladder regularly or take a quick nap.

Or just embrace it for what it is. If it makes others uncomfortable, well, join the club! Plus, why be ashamed of a natural process? Be who you are, face what you're facing without shame, and if anyone has a problem with that, it's on them.

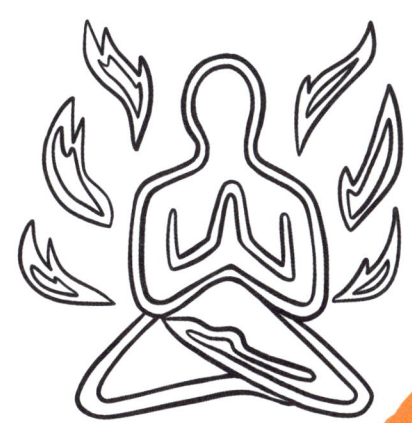

MENOPAUSE MYTH BUSTERS: SORTING FACT FROM FICTION

Test your meno-knowledge with this quiz. For each question, only one answer is correct. Can you figure out which one it is?

1. **The first sign of perimenopause is:**
   a. Jekyll and Hyde syndrome
   b. Irregular menstrual cycles
   c. Gaining the perimenopause fifteen
   d. Narcolepsy during boring work meetings

2. **Earlier onset menopause may be due to:**
   a. Your "it's five o'clock somewhere" cocktail routine
   b. Smoking ciggies
   c. More than two pregnancies—so many hormones!
   d. Being the first to "develop" of your friends

3. **Hot flashes:**
   a. Can be triggered by tight clothing; we're looking at you, skinny jeans
   b. Are not able to be controlled, except through medication
   c. Tend to be more frequent after sleeping in
   d. Are best dealt with by having chocolate and wine, yes please!

4. **Up to 90 percent of women:**
   a. Experience hot flashes
   b. Reach menopause by age fifty
   c. Gain weight after menopause
   d. Have minimal symptoms

5. **Menopause can bring many weird changes to your body. The following is NOT known to be one of them (don't say we don't give you good news sometimes!):**
   a. Tinnitus
   b. Electric shocks
   c. Bronchitis
   d. Burning tongue

6. **Perimenopause typically lasts for:**
   a. A mere eighteen months—you got this!
   b. Four years, give or take
   c. So that's why they call it the seven-year itch
   d. Fourteen years; this is a sick joke

7. **You get your toaster for having officially reached menopause when:**
   a. You have your first hot flash
   b. You have your first irregular period
   c. You haven't had a period for twelve months
   d. You hit fifty years old

8. **The average hot flash lasts for:**
   a. 20 seconds
   b. 4 minutes
   c. 10 minutes
   d. Who cares what my watch says, it's an eternity!

9. **During a hot flash:**
   a. Blood vessels near the skin contract
   b. Eyes dry out and get itchy
   c. The heart slows down
   d. The heart speeds up

10. **Apart from people, which other mammal goes through menopause?**
    a. Elephants
    b. Chimpanzees
    c. Orcas
    d. Beavers

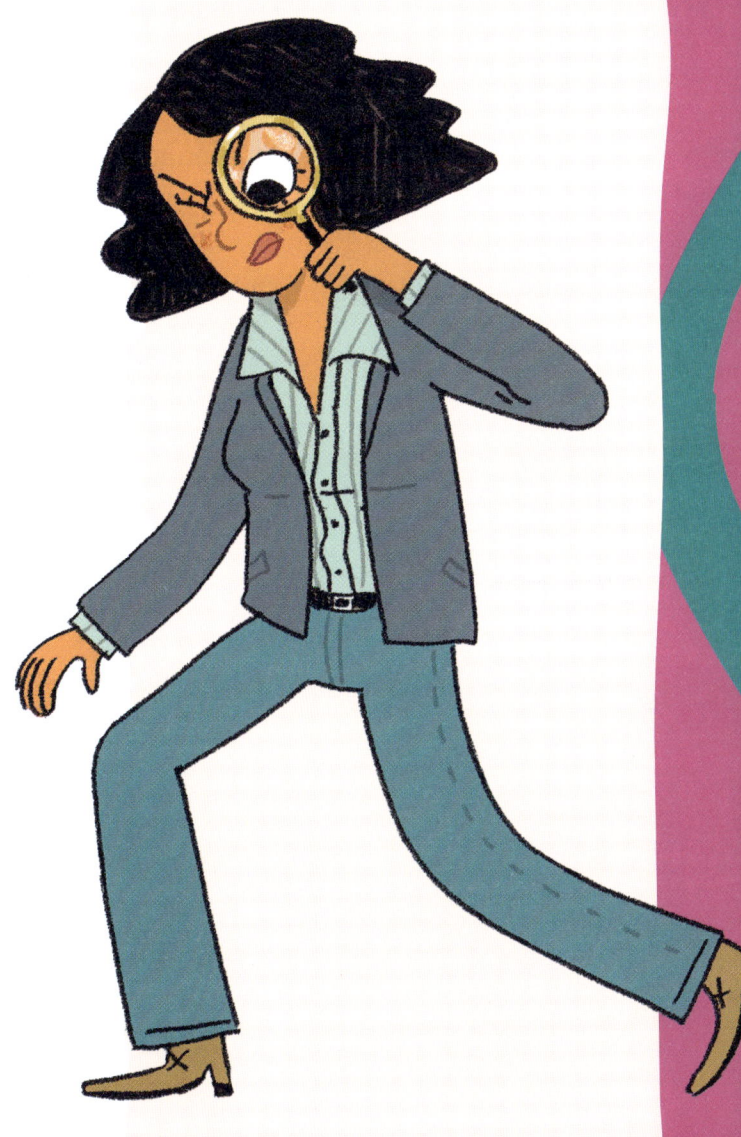

Answers on page 92.

YOU AND ME, BABE

How are you handling this phase of life? Time to get someone else's opinion! Ask your partner or bestie these questions about yourself, and then fill in their answers in the blanks below to create a little story, all about you!

1. What menopause symptom do you think is hardest for me? _____

2. What is something I keep with me at all times? _____

3. What annoys me? _____

4. What is my guilty pleasure? _____

5. What other menopausal symptoms do you think I get? List as many as you can.
_____, _____, _____

6. If I could go for a holiday anywhere, where would I go? _____

7. What would I do there? _____

8. What do I appreciate most about YOU (the bestie/partner)?
_____

9. What is something you enjoy doing with me? _____

10. How would you describe my personality? _____

Now, fill in their answers to write your story! You may need to change the grammar of answers your partner or bestie gave slightly to make them fit into the story structure.

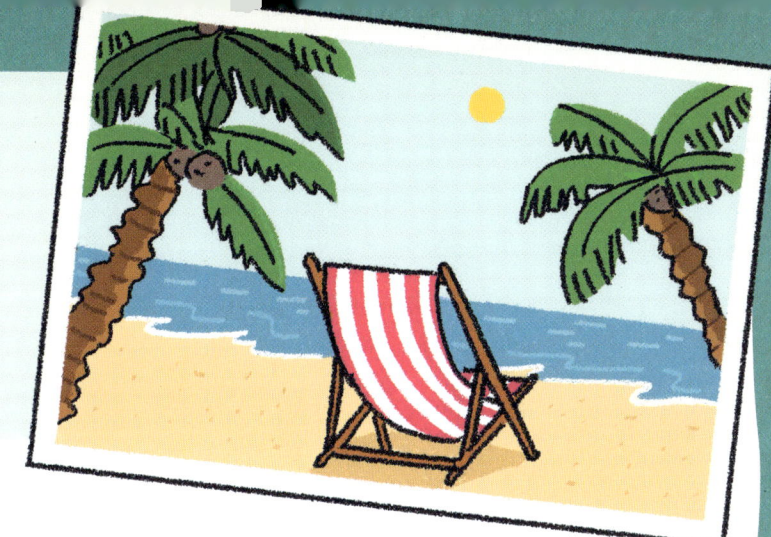

When _____ gets a _____ ,
(insert your name)   (insert answer to number 1)

she reaches for her _____ . Unless she can't find it,
(insert answer to number 2)

which happens more and more often these days! This is almost as annoying as

_____ , so to feel better, she_____ .
(insert answer to number 3)   (insert answer to number 4)

On tough days, when she is hit with _____ , she dreams of
(insert answer to number 5)

escaping to _____ to _____ .
(insert answer to number 6)   (insert answer to number 7)

But then reality hits, so instead, she finds_____ ,
(insert partner or bestie's name)

who is_____ . Together, they _____ ,
(insert answer to number 8)   (insert answer to number 9)

which makes her feel_____ .
(insert answer to number 10)

Dealing with menopause isn't so bad after all, with you along for the ride!

BY ANY OTHER NAME

Menopause and Perimenopause and their common symptoms have been called many different names. Oh yes, the poets have been busy. Find these alternate names in the word search below.

INTERNAL FURNACE

PERSONAL SUMMER

OVARIAN RETIREMENT

POWER SURGE

REVERSE PUBERTY

SECOND SPRING

NIGHTCRAWLERS

SUPER-SOAKER EVENT

CLOSED BABY FACTORY

THE CHANGE

THE SWITCH

MURDERPAUSE

VICTORIA'S SECRET

HELLAPAUSE

GLAND FINALE

HYPER PUBERTY

MENTALPAUSE

TEMPERATURE TANTRUM

INTERNAL RESET

OVARY OVERHAUL

```
P E R S O N A L S U M M E R I L O K U I N
I N T E R N A L R E S E T J T C V T I N M
O V A R Y O V E R H A U L E R L A E D T E
S Z Z N T P O W E R S U R G E O R M K E L
U C O V Y G P I P B T C A D V S I P S R I
P K H Y P E R P U B E R T Y E E A E Q N L
E N T H M U P K K S E T D I R D N R R A N
R P H B D X Q J S S J H K Q S B R A M L I
S V E Z R U C A U Q G E D H E A E T E F G
O H W R F A I A A M L C S Z P B T U N U H
A B K F R R P I A U A H E C U Y I R T R T
K O G P O A F B H R N A C E B F R E A N C
E O C T L P G C Z D D N O N E A E T L A R
R L C L X X T E J E F G N Z R C M A P C A
E I E U D I Q N A R I E D F T T E N A E W
V H Y V W H E U I P N I S U Y O N T U U L
E N S S B J N F R A A B P I M R T R S K E
N S E A E G M U S U L T R Z G Y S U E N R
T H W I R L N T N S E F I K E W S M N D S
T C R O I B M A E E I N N G O E P B H B H
X M D H H Q G G V X T I G H U H A E K R T
```

Answers on page 92.

22

STOP THE LEAKS MAZE!

Once upon a time, our bladders were made of steel and did our bidding. Nowadays, they are more like water balloons, and when it's time to go, they'll explode all over everything. Fight your way through this maze avoiding all the inconvenient places you now feel the need to pee!

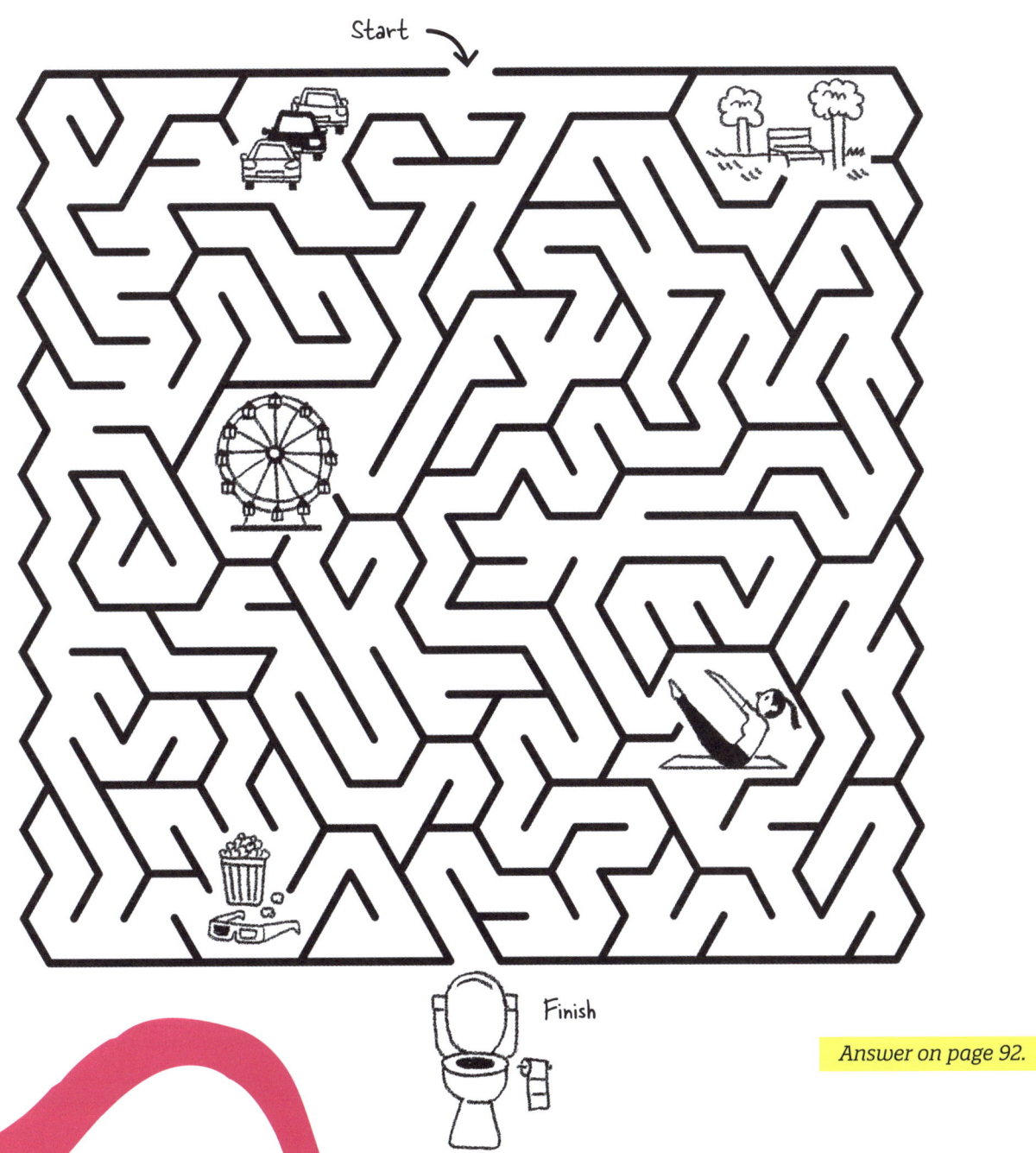

Start

Finish

Answer on page 92.

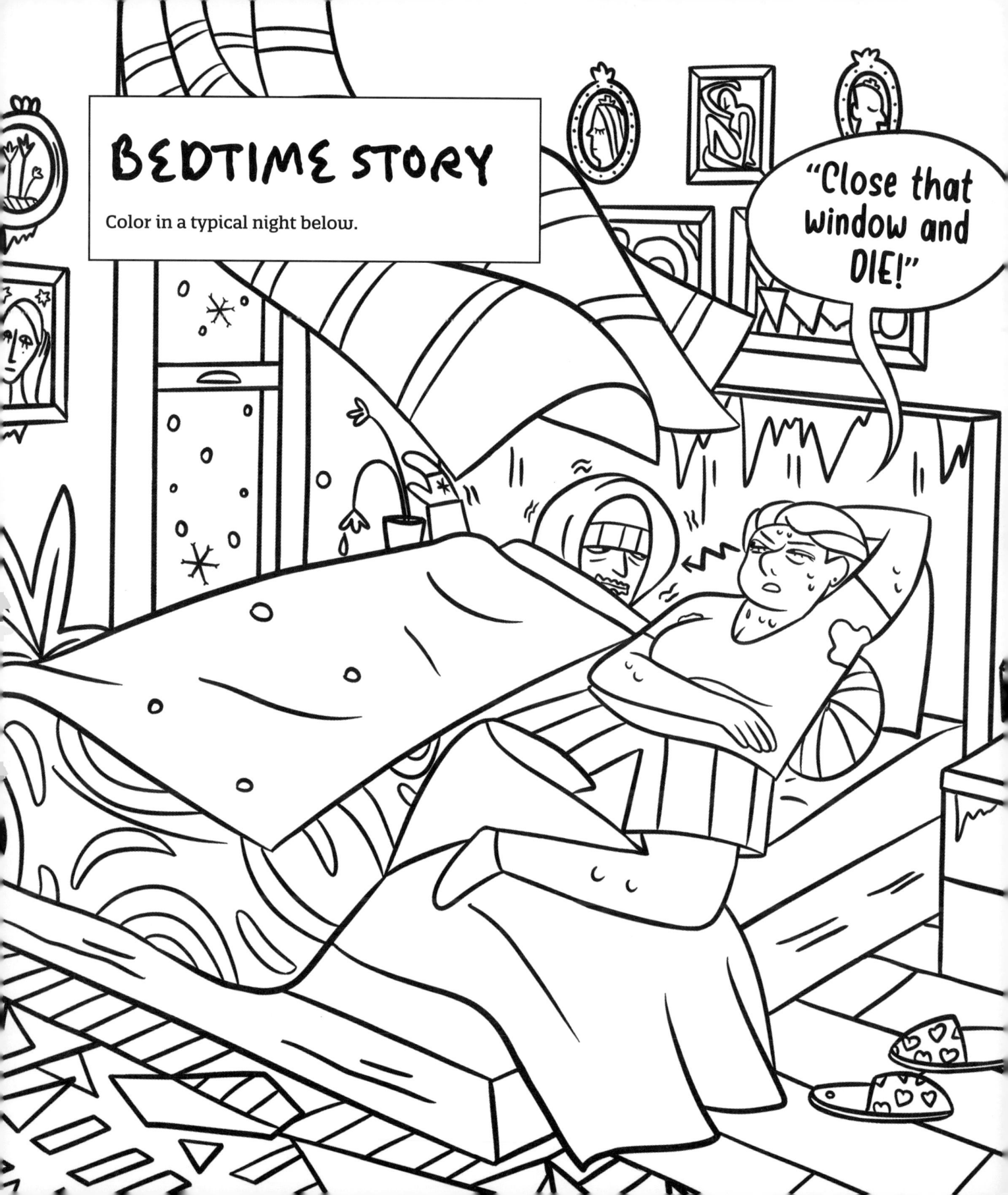

MENOPAUSE MARQUEE

Margaret Mead (1901–1978), an American cultural anthropologist, said some wise words about menopause. We want the world to know it, so we have put it up on a sign, with lights! Unfortunately, some of the letters have fallen off. Place them back in the right spots to rebuild the sign and see this quote yourself.

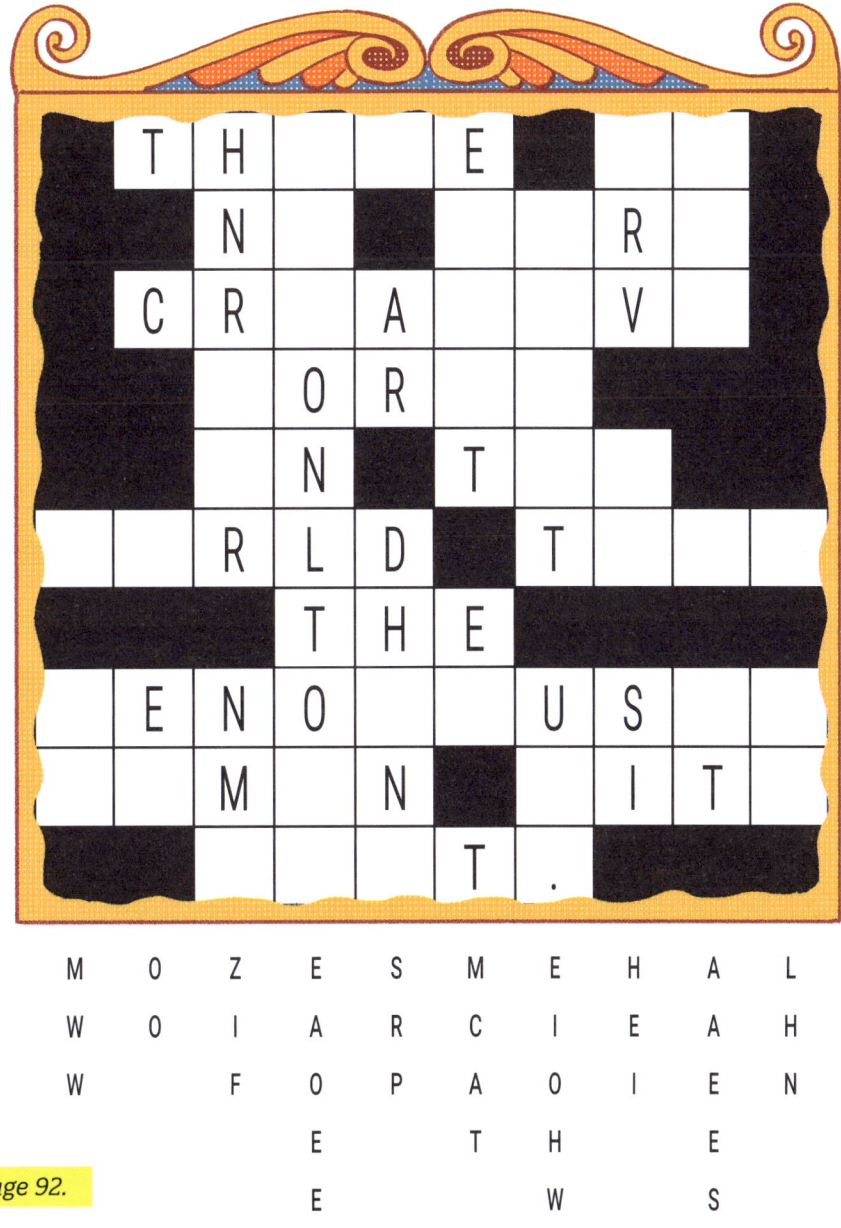

M	O	Z	E	S	M	E	H	A	L
W	O	I	A	R	C	I	E	A	H
W		F	O	P	A	O	I	E	N
		E		T	H			E	
		E		W				S	

Answer on page 92.

TRICKY TERMINOLOGY

Do you know these tricky menopause terms? Improve your lexicon and sound like a proper expert by finding the correct definition for each of these words.

1. **Oogenesis**
   a. The act of staring intently at others to try and discern whether they are facing the same problems as the viewer, for example, scrutinizing someone to detect the onset of a hot flash
   b. The production of egg cells, which ends with menopause
   c. The name of an all-female rock band
   d. The first time you notice pain associated with vaginal dryness during sex

2. **Climacteric**
   a. The exact point at which a mood swings
   b. An environment conducive to lovemaking. Candles and Prince, anyone? Or just some good lube?
   c. The time of life when fertility is at a decline, a synonym for menopause
   d. When it feels far too hot, no matter how many windows are open or fans are running; or when it feels far too cold, even when heaters or fires are running at full throttle

3. **Psychoneuroendocrinology**
   a. Field of research that studies how hormones can impact mental illness
   b. Medical term for the graying of eyebrow hairs
   c. Neurological treatment for menopausal symptoms, as opposed to hormonal treatment
   d. Burgeoning study of criminal tendencies that manifest during perimenopause

4. **Osteopenia**
   a. Sensitive teeth with a metallic taste in the mouth, a rarer menopausal symptom
   b. Loss of bone mineral density, which often occurs during menopause
   c. Poor posture as a result of aging and hormonal changes
   d. Loss of pelvic floor strength, resulting in lots of pee

5. **Progesterone**
   a. Hormone that prepares the lining of the uterus for an egg to grow
   b. Being supportive of steroid use
   c. Lower back pain
   d. Movement advocating for the abolishment of bras

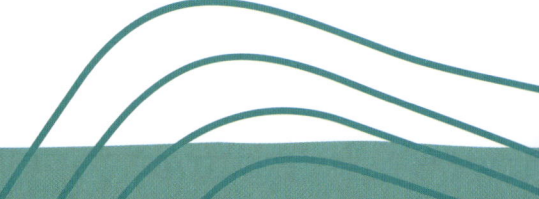

6. **POI**
   a. Point Of Indifference—when you just don't give a shit anymore
   b. Personal Oven Ignition—you're so hot right now
   c. Peeing Overload Intensification—when a bladder seems perpetually full, to the point of bursting
   d. Premature Ovarian Insufficiency—loss of ovarian function in those younger than forty

7. **HRT**
   a. Hormonal Roller-coaster Time—the peak of moodiness during menopause, and a time for utmost caution for those nearby
   b. Hormone Replacement Therapy—used to alleviate estrogen deficiency symptoms
   c. Hairy, Roasting, Tired—basically, leave me alone
   d. Hirsutism Reduction Treatments—dealing with unwanted hair

8. **Telogen Effluvium**
   a. State of lethargy, regularly occurring in perimenopause
   b. Ability to remember complicated TV series plots, but not where you put your keys
   c. Hair loss, often due to hormonal imbalance
   d. Nausea and dizziness, especially when getting up quickly

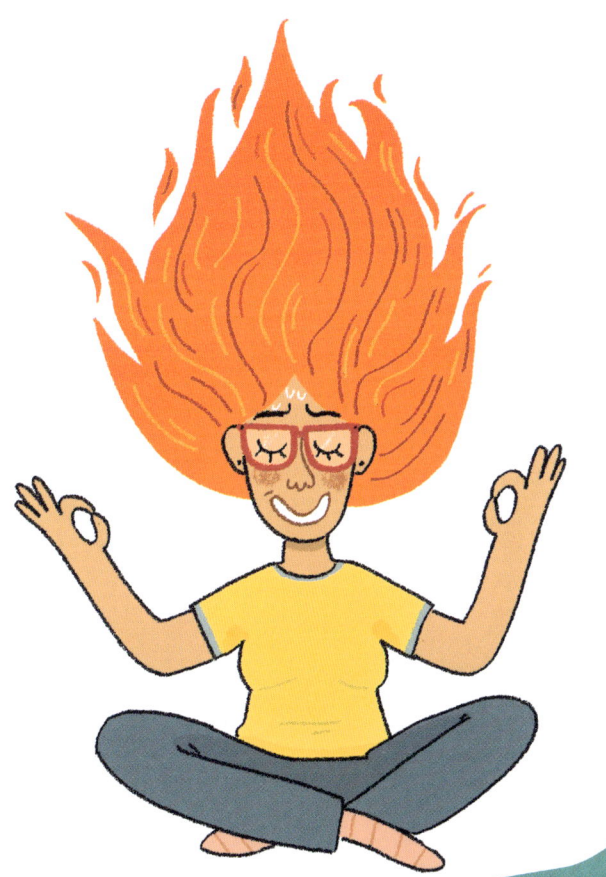

Answers on page 93.

HOLDING TIGHT AND LETTING GO

Inside your hands, draw or write all the things you want to hold tightly as you go through this stage of life. It might be certain people, goals or dreams you have, or assurances that you don't want to forget when times are bumpy.

On the outside of your hands, draw or write all the things you are letting go of. Some things you may not have a choice about, as your body changes. Others might be more of a personal decision to leave behind or stop working toward. When you're done, color this in and look back on it.

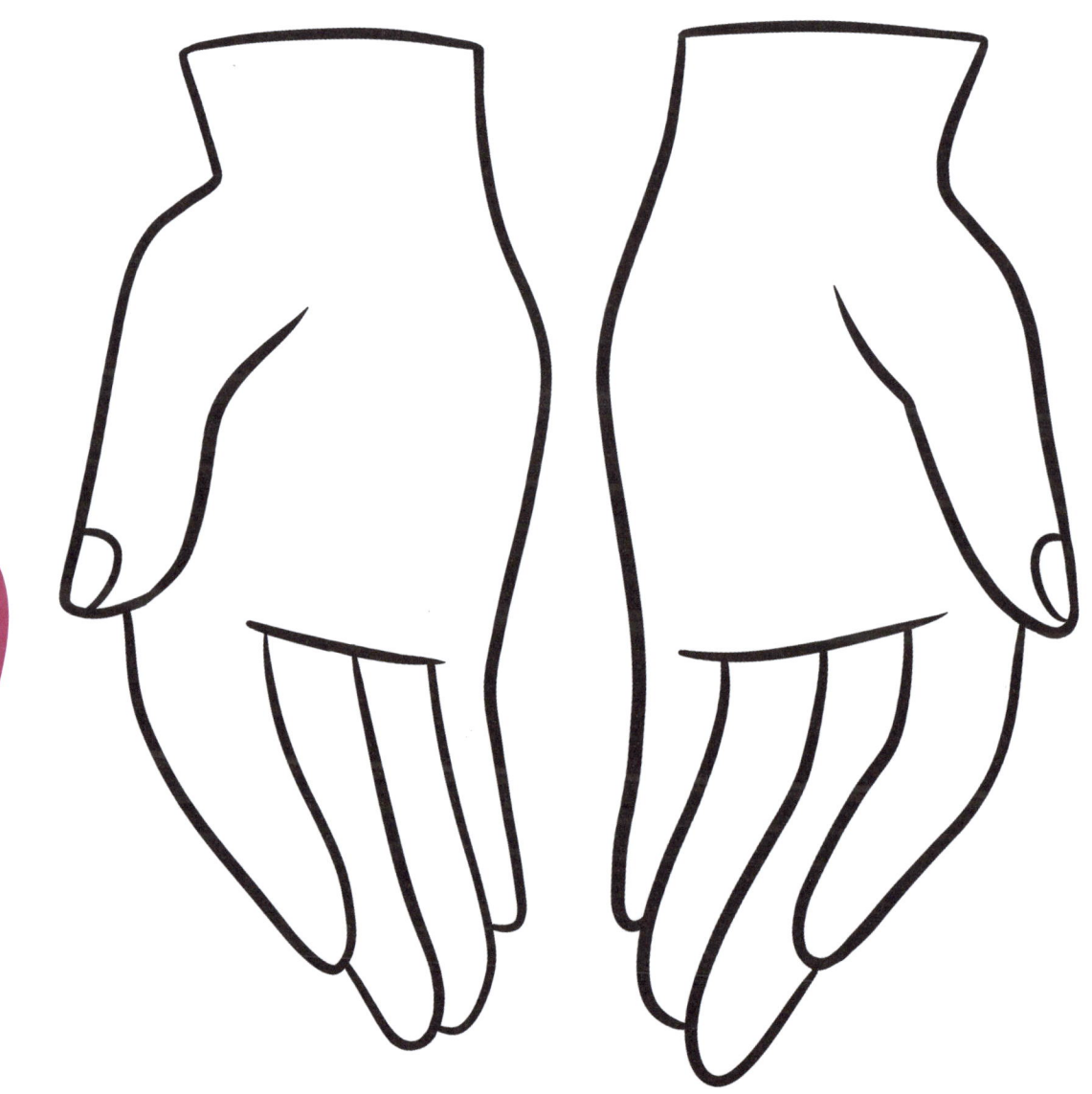

MENOPAUSAL SCRABBLE

Use the letters in MENOPAUSAL to find as many words as you can. How many points did you manage to get in the end?

1–2 letters
(2 points per word):

AM
UP

_____

_____

_____

_____

_____

_____

_____

_____

3 letters
(3 points per word):

MOP
SPA

_____

_____

_____

_____

_____

_____

_____

_____

4 letters
(4 points per word):

OMEN
NOPE

_____

_____

_____

_____

_____

_____

_____

_____

5 letters
(5 points per word):

SALON
MAULS

_____

_____

_____

_____

_____

_____

6 or more letters
(10 points per word):

SAMPLE
SUNLAMP

_____

_____

_____

_____

_____

_____

TOTAL POINTS

_____

M
E
N
O
P
A
U
S
A
L

SHAKESPEAREAN MIC DROPS: PART I

No, the Bard himself never underwent menopause, but, as a keen observer of human character, Shakespeare had a lot to say that we can relate to this phase of life. Next time someone asks you how you're doing, refer to these handy quotes and fire one off dramatically for maximum impact. If you're crafty, why not embroider and decorate your favorite quote to display?

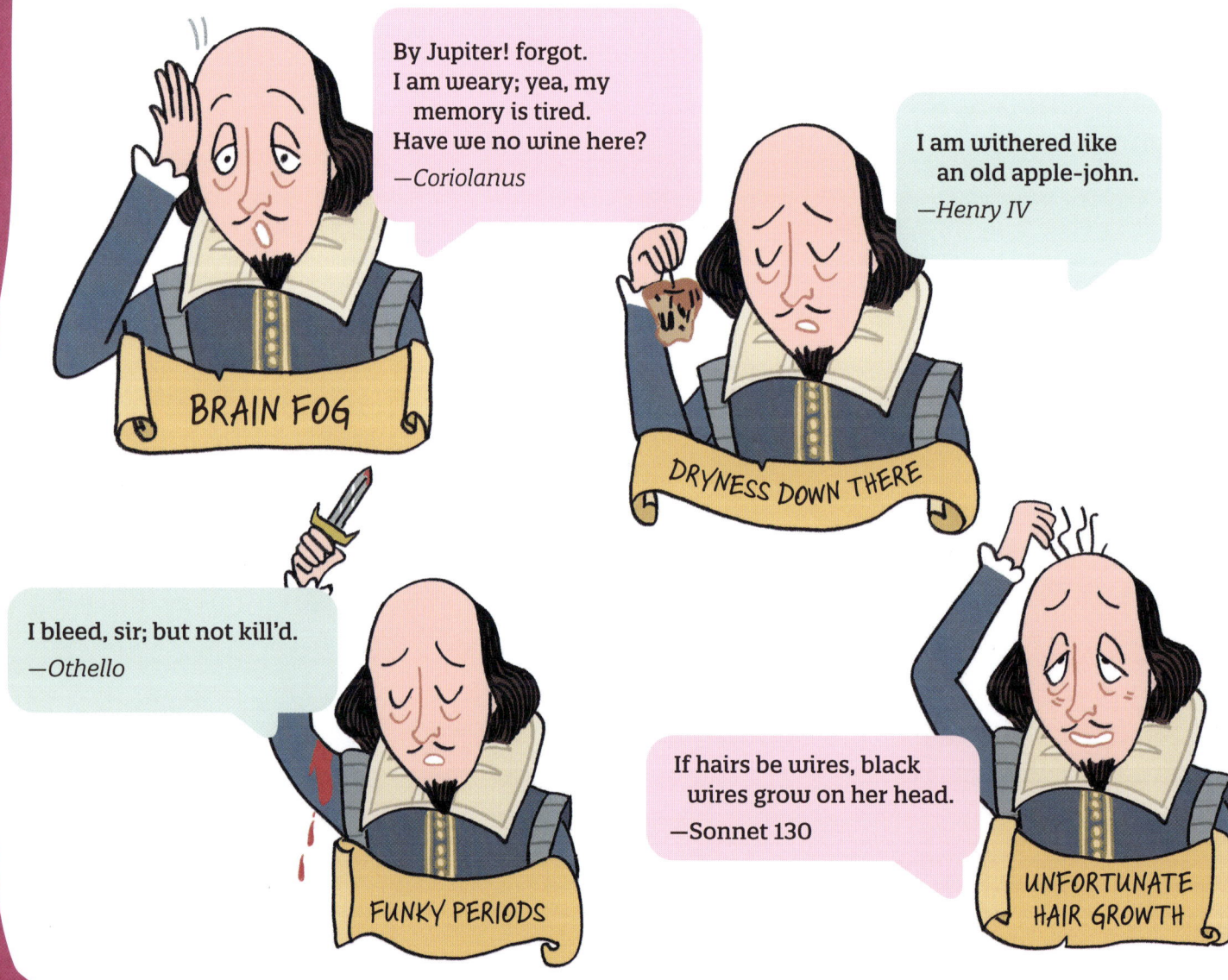

By Jupiter! forgot.
I am weary; yea, my memory is tired.
Have we no wine here?
—*Coriolanus*

BRAIN FOG

I am withered like an old apple-john.
—*Henry IV*

DRYNESS DOWN THERE

I bleed, sir; but not kill'd.
—*Othello*

FUNKY PERIODS

If hairs be wires, black wires grow on her head.
—Sonnet 130

UNFORTUNATE HAIR GROWTH

But age, with his stealing steps,
Hath claw'd me in his clutch,
And hath shipped me into the land,
As if I had never been such.

—*Hamlet*

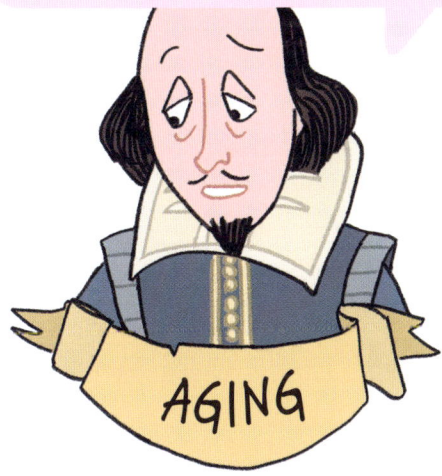

AGING

Women will all turn monsters.

—*King Lear*

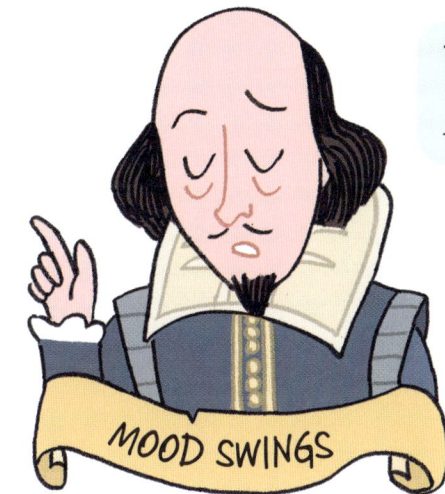

MOOD SWINGS

Let us seek out some desolate shade, and there
Weep our sad bosoms empty.

—*Macbeth*

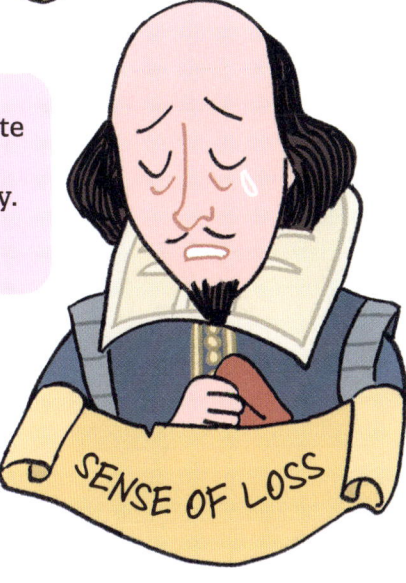

SENSE OF LOSS

But, woe is me, you are so sick of late,
So far from cheer and from your former state,

—*Hamlet*

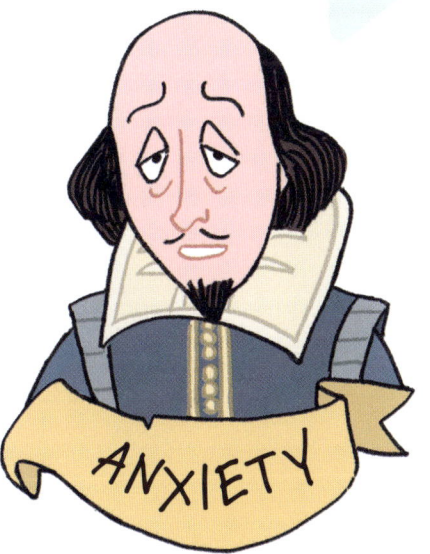

ANXIETY

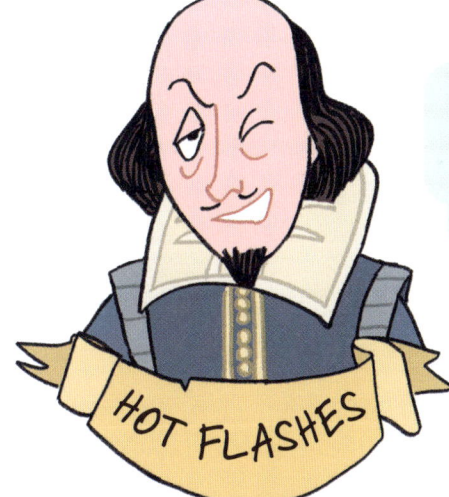

HOT FLASHES

Is she so hot a shrew as she's reported?

—*The Taming of the Shrew*

HORMONAL POWDER KEG

Big props to those who share their lives with teenagers. You're not just dealing with your own wild hormonal rides but having to cope with theirs as well. There are sure to be sparks and, occasionally, explosions. Search for all the shared symptoms of puberty and perimenopause.

ATTITUDE

CRAMPS

SASS

IT'S NOT FAIR

BRAIN FOG

CRYING

PIMPLES

MOODY

CHANGES

ESTROGEN

INSOMNIA

GROWTH

HORMONES

PERIODS

TANTRUMS

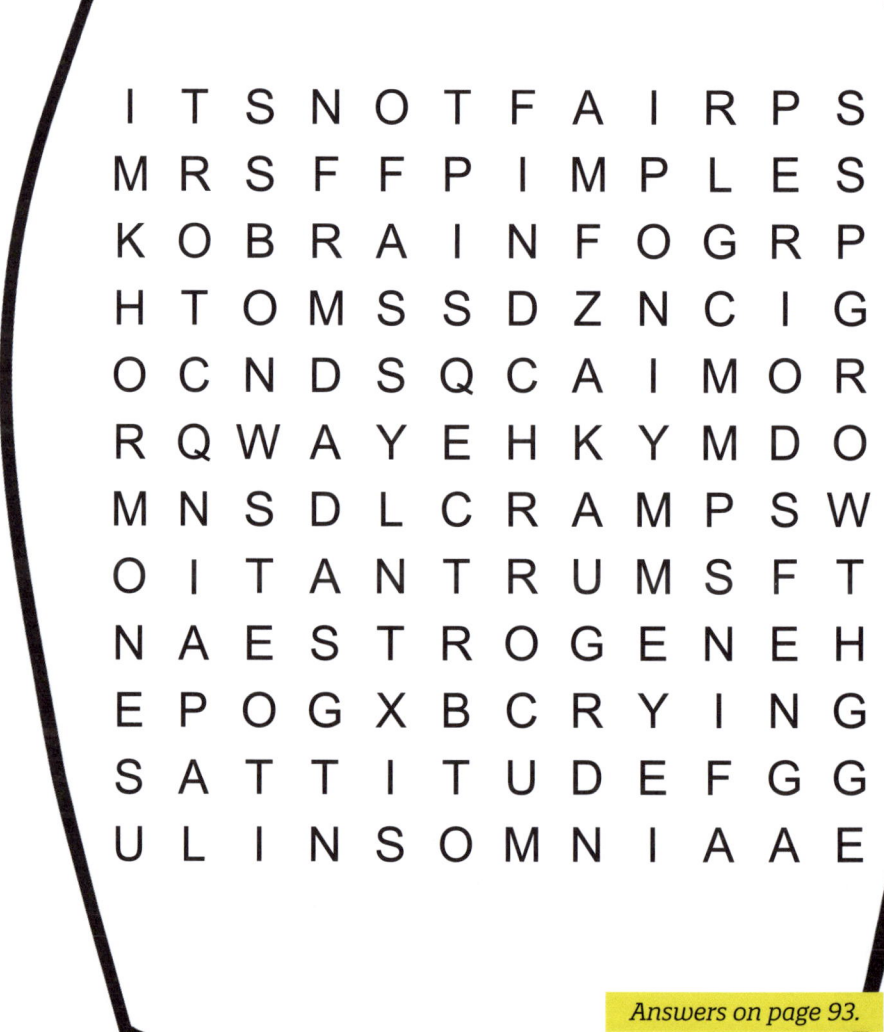

```
I T S N O T F A I R P S
M R S F F P I M P L E S
K O B R A I N F O G R P
H T O M S S D Z N C I G
O C N D S Q C A I M O R
R Q W A Y E H K Y M D O
M N S D L C R A M P S W
O I T A N T R U M S F T
N A E S T R O G E N E H
E P O G X B C R Y I N G
S A T T I T U D E F G G
U L I N S O M N I A A E
```

Answers on page 93.

WHERE DID I PUT MY KEYS?

Your brain isn't your womb, so why does perimenopause seem to be shutting it down as well? Welcome to brain fog. It doesn't matter how switched on you are, chances are, you'll also have to rack your brain one day to find your keys . . . or phone . . . or house! Follow the maze to search your entire place—*is it in the fridge? did I throw it away? in the flowerpot?*—and find out where you left your keys this time . . .

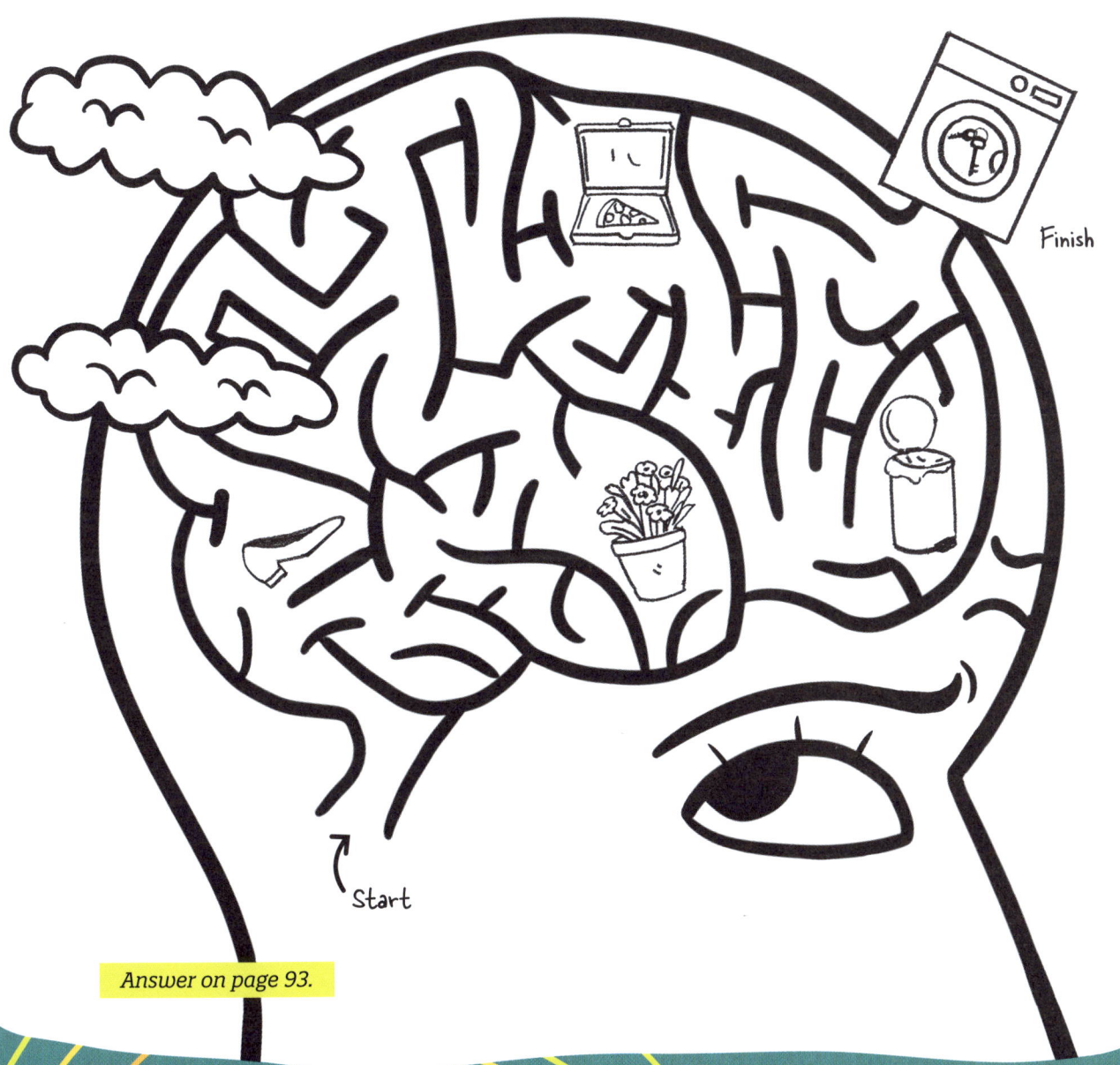

Start

Finish

Answer on page 93.

SNAKES AND LADDERS OF MENOPAUSE

The Change is full of ups and downs. Play a friend or challenge yourself to see whether you can survive unscathed. You will need a die and counters for all who play. Start at number 1 and see who is the first to make it to Menopause at the end—go up the ladders and slide down the snakes!

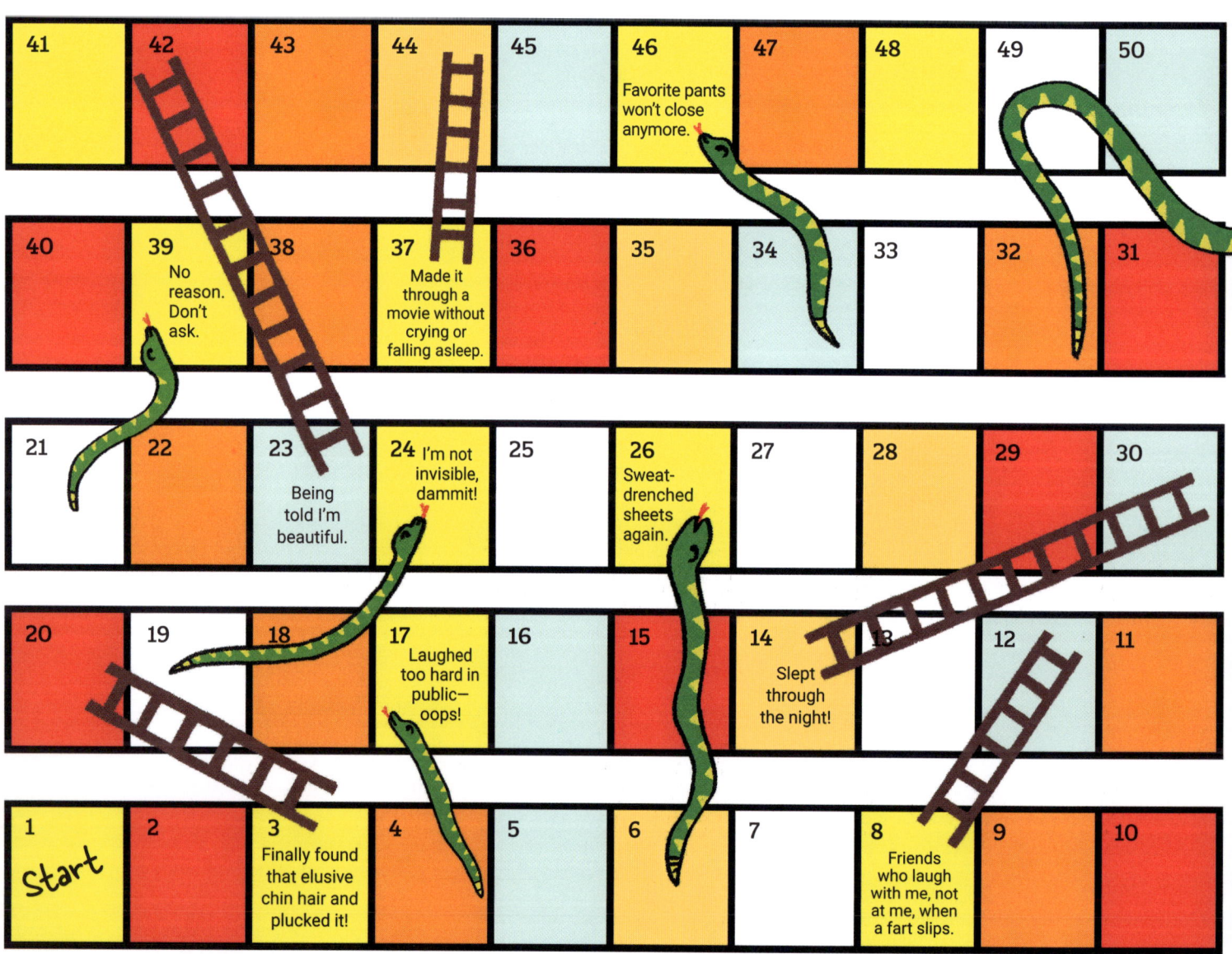

41	42	43	44	45	46 Favorite pants won't close anymore.	47	48	49	50
40	39 No reason. Don't ask.	38	37 Made it through a movie without crying or falling asleep.	36	35	34	33	32	31
21	22	23 Being told I'm beautiful.	24 I'm not invisible, dammit!	25	26 Sweat-drenched sheets again.	27	28	29	30
20	19	18	17 Laughed too hard in public—oops!	16	15	14 Slept through the night!	13	12	11
1 Start	2	3 Finally found that elusive chin hair and plucked it!	4	5	6	7	8 Friends who laugh with me, not at me, when a fart slips.	9	10

Welcome to perimenopause!
Prepare for the wild ride ahead!

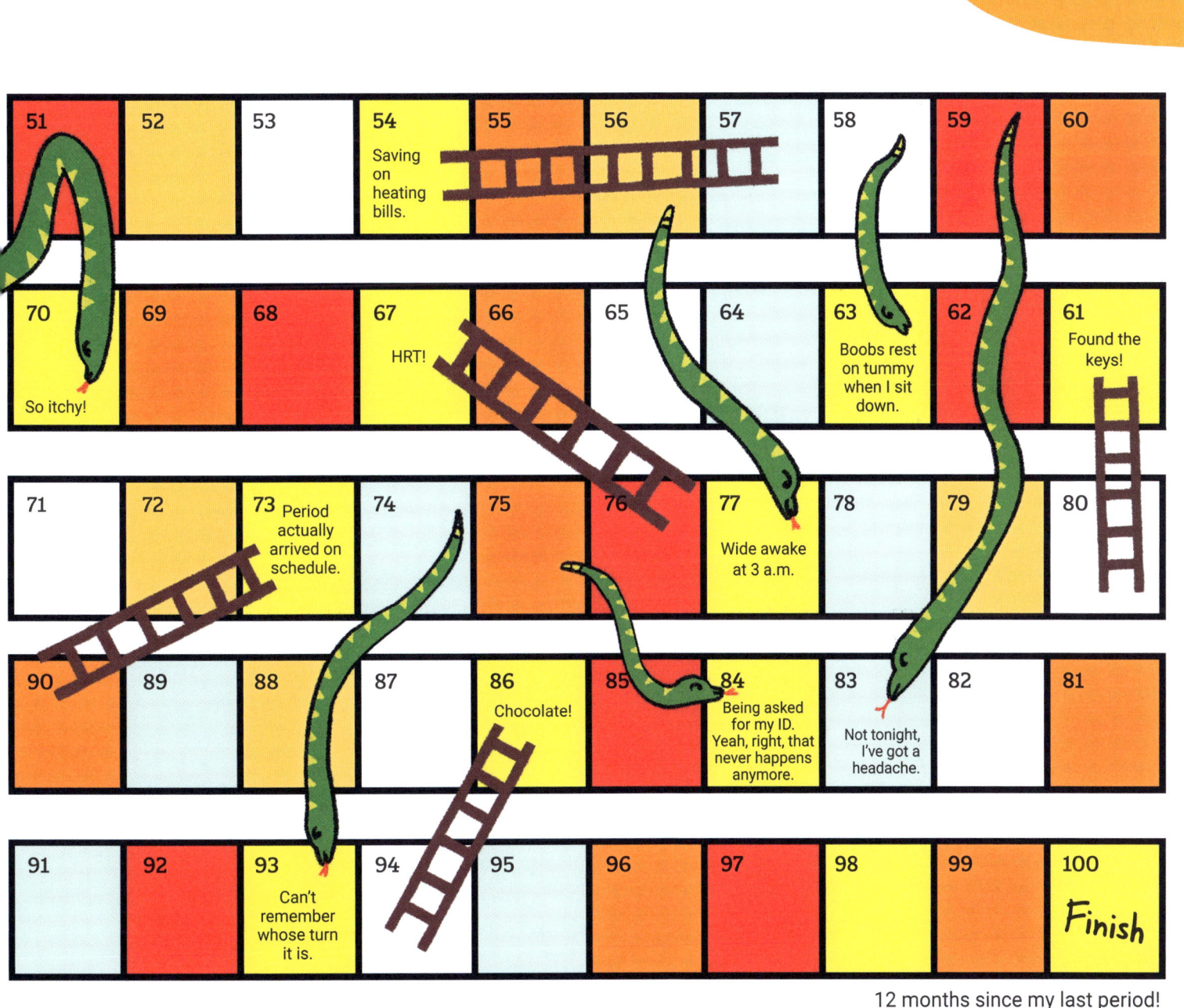

51	52	53	54 Saving on heating bills.	55	56	57	58	59	60
70 So itchy!	69	68	67 HRT!	66	65	64	63 Boobs rest on tummy when I sit down.	62	61 Found the keys!
71	72	73 Period actually arrived on schedule.	74	75	76	77 Wide awake at 3 a.m.	78	79	80
90	89	88	87	86 Chocolate!	85	84 Being asked for my ID. Yeah, right, that never happens anymore.	83 Not tonight, I've got a headache.	82	81
91	92	93 Can't remember whose turn it is.	94	95	96	97	98	99	100 Finish

12 months since my last period!
Menopause unlocked!

35

ME AND MY MENOPAUSE POEM

We all experience menopause in different ways. For each question, circle the answer that best describes you, then flip the page and fill it in the corresponding blank to make your customized menopause poem!

1. **My hair is:**
   - Luscious, flowing, thick, and wild
   - Sporadic, wiry, dull, and gray
   - Curly and untamable
   - Little, stubborn wires

2. **Best tip for dealing with a bulging tummy:**
   - Squeeze into tight shapewear
   - Hold my breath and suck in hard
   - Give up doing anything
   - Wear medieval corsets

3. **To mitigate the risk of accidental bladder leakage, I:**
   - Keep maps of restrooms in my town
   - Put leakproof adult diapers on
   - Refuse to laugh before I've peed
   - Keep my legs crossed each time I laugh

4. **I look in the mirror and see:**
   - Exhausted eyes, new laughter lines
   - Blotchy, oily, zitty skin
   - I look just like my mother now
   - A resting bitch, am I a witch?

5. **What is unreliable?**
   - Printers, always breaking down
   - Trains that never come on time
   - Mail, expected months ago
   - Perfect weather forecasts

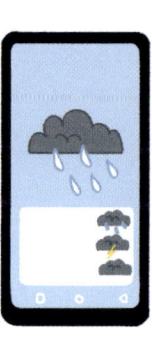

6. **I relax in:**
   - Tracksuit pants with loose waistbands
   - Baggy vests that let me sweat
   - So many layers, on and off
   - Pajamas and high-waisted pants

7. **I really hate:**
   - Hot flashes, sweats, and stinky breath
   - Being called "ma'am," getting offered seats
   - Being ignored or called a "Karen"
   - These wild banshees that live in me

8. **It's date night! What's different these days?**
   - Back home at nine, then sleeping time
   - Shapewear replaces lingerie
   - Fall asleep at the theater
   - I cry, regardless of the film

9. **What makes me laugh?**
   - I accidentally slip a fart
   - A guy says, "I know how you feel"
   - My partner asks, "You in the mood?"
   - "So, did you have a good sleep?"

10. **I have been most likely to forget:**
   - What I was doing next
   - To turn the oven off
   - The place I put my keys
   - Each of my children's names

11. **Biggest turn-ons:**
   - My honey does their sexy move
   - Jason Momoa rips his shirt
   - Soft jazz is playing, candles lit
   - A hot massage, a steamy kiss

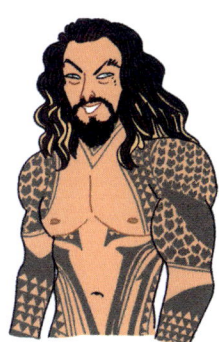

12. **Things I can't do now:**
   - Regulate my mood swings
   - Get wolf whistles anymore
   - Stay awake to watch a film
   - Wear the size I used to

13. **What a hot flash is like:**
   - Swimming in a volcano
   - Being stuck inside a sauna
   - Spontaneous combustion
   - Being plunged into the depths of Hell

14. **What I do now that I never would have before:**
   - Will not take shit anymore
   - Live in my pajama pants
   - Say "no" with more confidence
   - Eat more chocolate, drink more wine

15. **In one day, I can feel:**
   - Dizzy, grumpy, anxious
   - Clammy, cold, irritable
   - Sleepy, itchy, forgetful
   - Nauseous, frigid, hopeless

16. **A sure way to annoy me is to:**
   - Turn the A/C off
   - Ask if I've gained weight
   - Say, "Get over it"
   - Say it's in my mind

17. **I am most excited about reaching menopause because:**
   - No cramps or periods
   - Sex without pregnancy
   - My hormones will align
   - My calm self will return

18. **I don't like how society can see me as:**
   - Invisible, irrelevant
   - Out to complain, I'm not a bitch
   - A has-been or a laughingstock
   - Embarrassing or past my prime

19. **I miss having:**
   - Sexy, perky boobs
   - Baby-making bits
   - Days of turning heads
   - Skimpy underthings

20. **The menopausal symptom I can't wait to be rid of the most is:**
   - Fear
   - Pain
   - Sweat
   - Moods

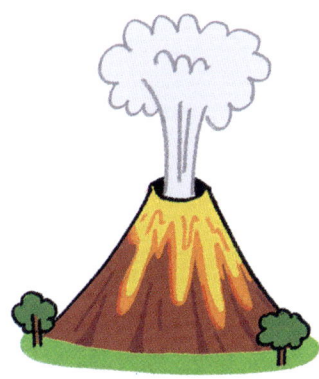

YOU'RE A POET AND YOU DIDN'T EVEN KNOW IT!

Take each of the answers you have chosen on the previous page and write them in the corresponding spaces in the poem below. Shakespeare has nothing on you, girl!

_____ — hair sprouting from my chin
1

_____ to keep my tummy in
2

_____ — I'm careful, "just in case"
3

_____ — what's happened to my face?
4

Like _____ my period comes and goes
5

_____ are my new favorite clothes
6

_____ — new things I really hate
7

_____ when I'm out on a date
8

_____. I laugh. Oops, was that pee?
9

Forgot _____. What's happening to me?
10

_____ — meh, down below's still dry

Can't _____ — it makes me want to cry

Like _____ — my thermostat's impaired

I _____ — before, I wouldn't dare!

_____ — all things I've felt today

And if you _____ , it's best to stay away!

But soon, _____ — there is that pot of gold

And I am not _____ or old

Okay, my _____ are gone; I let that go

And flush my _____

away—goodbye—no more, just like Aunt Flo!

39

HOWLING AT THE MOON

We are creatures with cycles, like the moon. When these get messed up, we might want to howl. You've got this, Beautiful One. Color this page.

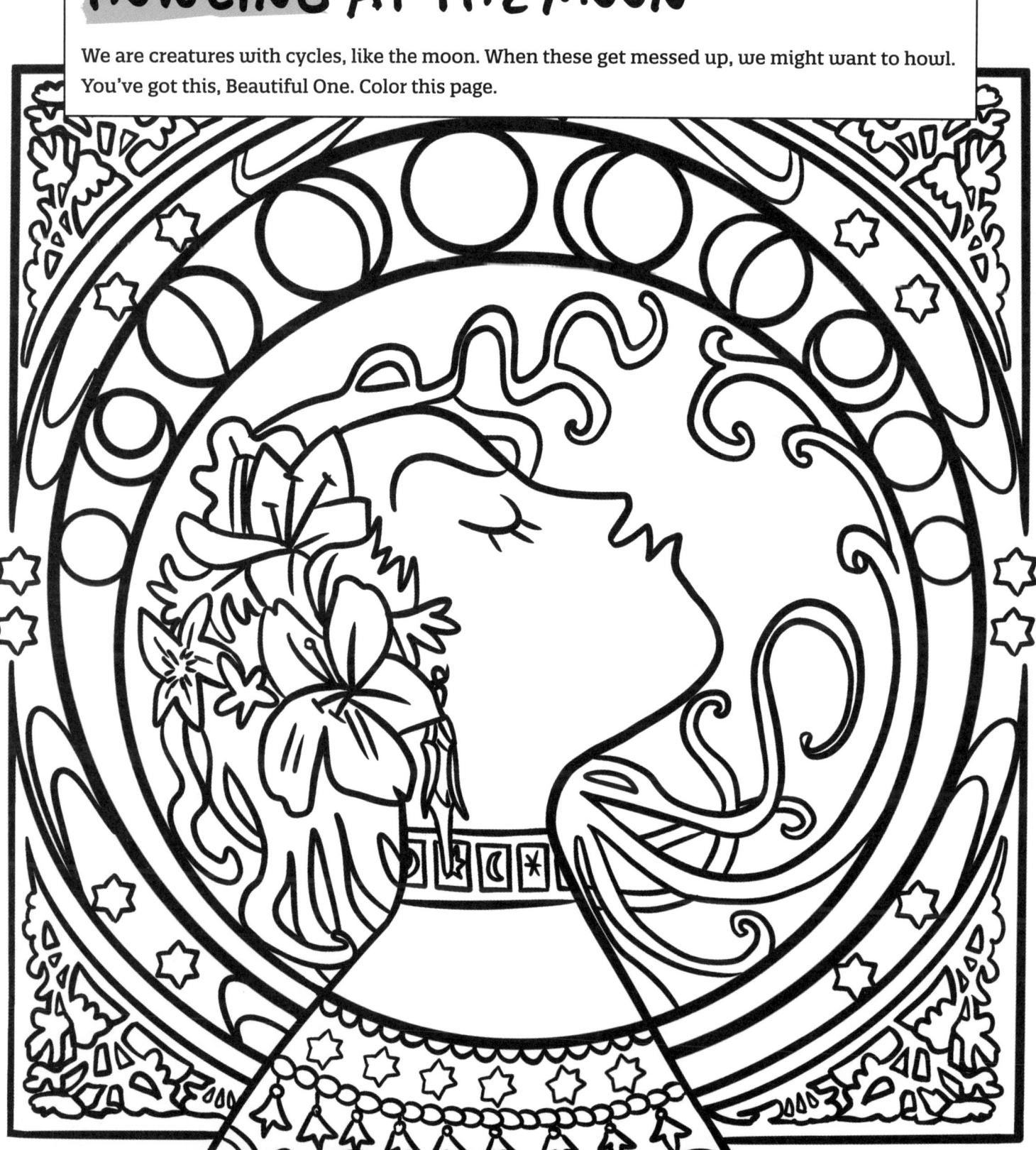

THE JOYS OF A WELL-PLACED FAN

Ever wonder why Marilyn Monroe looked so happy standing over the air vent? Perhaps she was having a perimenopausal hot flash! Connect the dots to reveal the picture.

NATURAL WAYS TO REDUCE SYMPTOMS

Many find relief through medication, and if that works for you, great! There are also some natural things you can do to help relieve perimenopausal discomfort, especially if they are habits in place before everything hits too hard. Complete the crossword puzzle to find a range of natural remedies available to you.

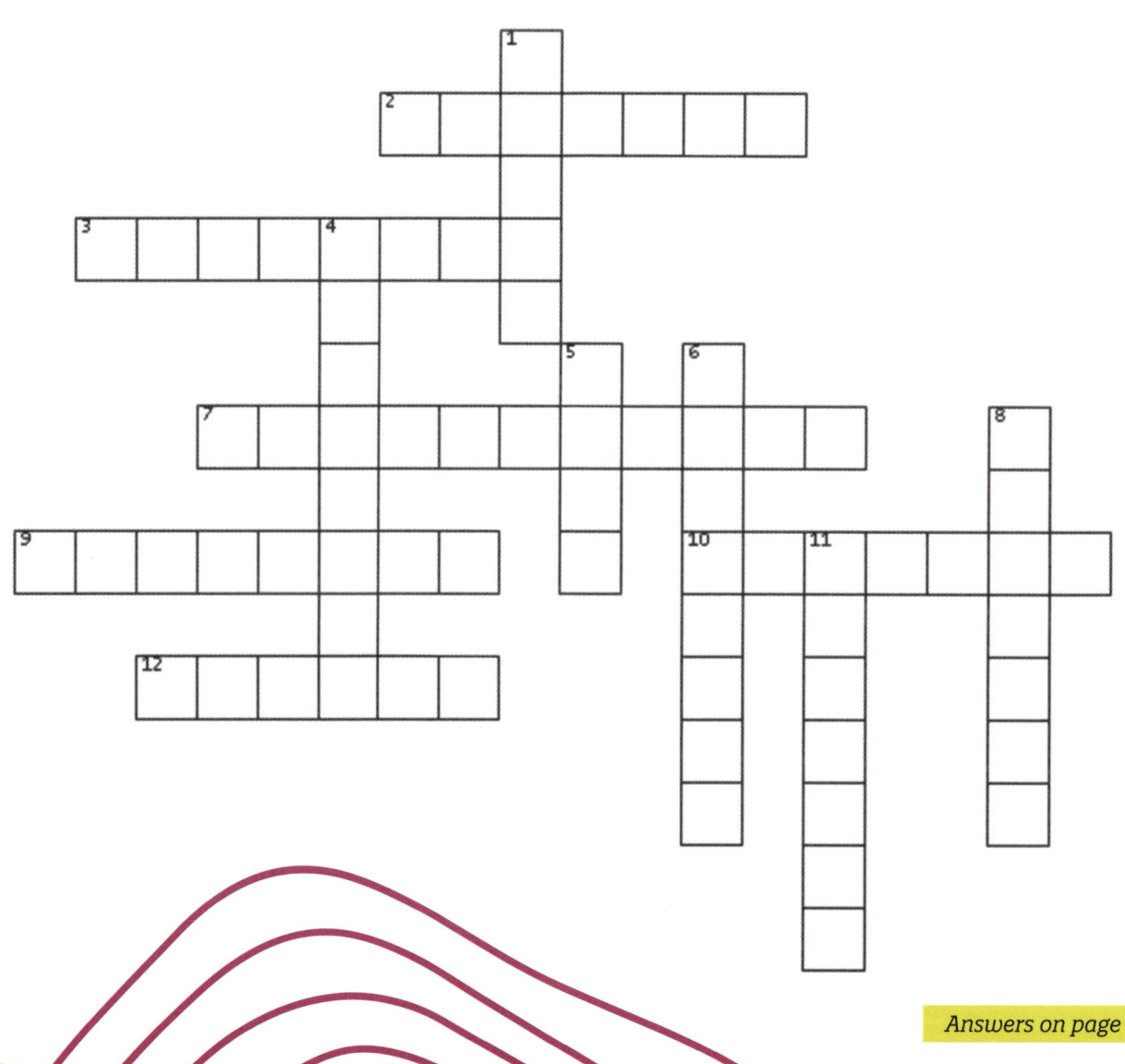

Answers on page 93.

ACROSS

2. A _____ diet helps you maintain weight. Unfortunately, the heavier we are, the more likely we are to get severe hot flashes. How unfair is that, seeing that weight gain is a menopausal "thing" too?!

3. Reduce _____ intake, as it can dehydrate you and bring on hot flashes. (Of course it might result in you feeling more zombie-like . . . a girl needs her coffee and chocolate, right?)

7. Sixty-six percent of respondents in a survey of six thousand people in menopause agreed that _____ is the most important way that everyone can support each other. Yes, it happens. Yes, it's okay to talk about. Yes, the bathroom is that way! (I'm next!)

9. Apply topical _____-_____ oil to the vagina for improved lubrication. It is thought to help with hot flashes as well. Just remember the letter (clue alert) to boost that excitement, eroticism, and energy!

10. Avoid drinking too much _____. It triggers menopausal symptoms and can result in poor sleep as well. Though some days, it may be worth it!

12. Meditate, go for walks, do yoga, or spend time in nature to reduce _____ levels. Or you might just need to ignore ACROSS clues 3 and 10, and just do what's best for you on the day, okay?

DOWN

1. Drink enough _____. This can help you maintain a healthy weight and reduce dryness symptoms.

4. Regular _____ can reduce mood swings and hot flashes, as well as minimize the risk of cardiovascular disease and help you sleep better.

5. Eat more foods that are _____ in phytoestrogens, like soy, tofu, beans, and flaxseeds. These are thought to reduce hot flashes and the risk of heart disease.

6. _____-_____ is considered to be the most valuable vitamin to take during menopause, because it helps bone health and lifts mood. So get out in the sun or eat some fish oil! Mmm!

8. No _____. I know. You know. But if you're looking for a more pressing reason to quit, studies show that those who quit or never started have a lower rate of hot flashes than those who still do this.

11. A good _____ intake helps strengthen your bones and improves general health. So pop some seeds, cheese, yogurt, and sardines! And maybe a little ice cream!

HOUSE PARTAY!

House parties between your twenties and now have too many differences to count! How many differences can you find in these two pictures?

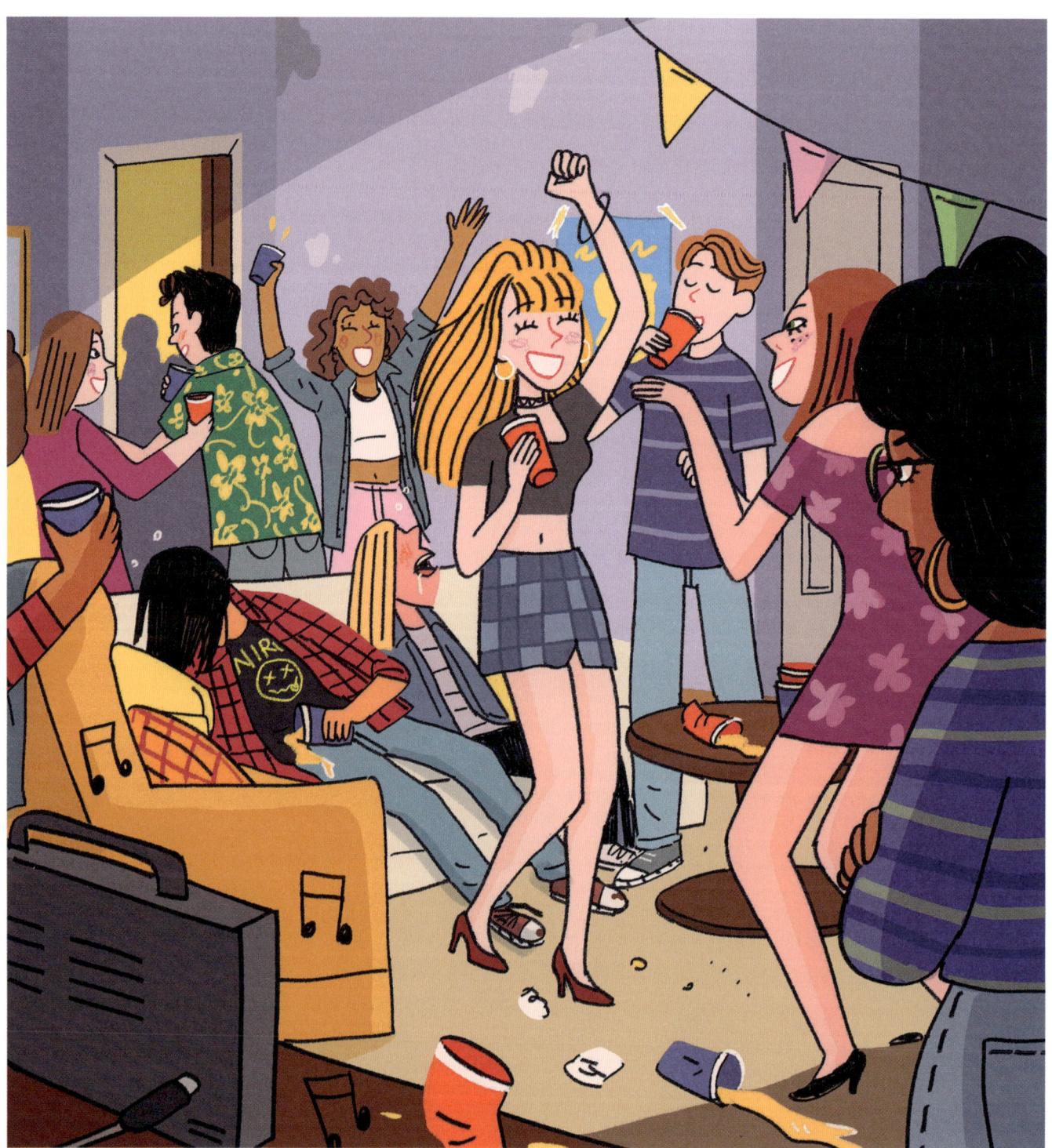

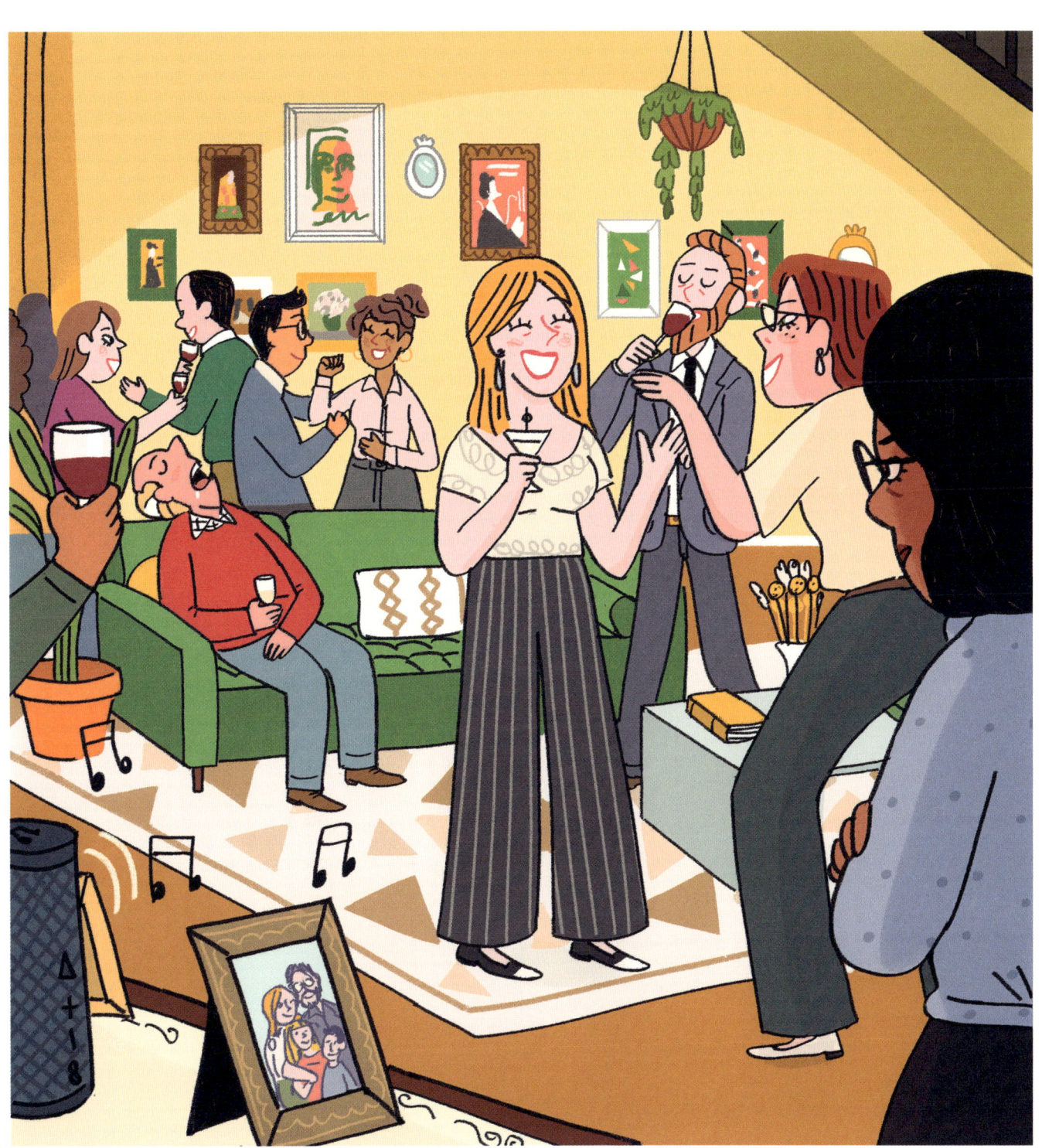

Answers on page 93.

BEAT THE BLAHS A TO Z

Use this A-to-Z list to help with ideas for managing perimenopausal blahs, from self-care to herbal remedies. *While these are all recommended by a variety of sources, it is always best to check with your health care provider first before adding new things to your diet or lifestyle, especially as some herbs are not as safe for those with preexisting conditions.*

A **Ashwagandha.** Also known as Indian ginseng or winter cherry, this herb is believed to help low mood, anxiety and fatigue, boost memory, and improve sleep.

B **B vitamins.** These serotonin boosters increase energy, fight depression, strengthen cognition, help with insomnia, and reduce hot flashes.

C **Coconut products.** Coconut oil moisturizes dry skin and conditions and strengthens hair. Add water and it can improve heart health and relax muscles, providing electrolytes, preventing fatigue, and boosting gut health.

D **Dancing.** Reduce stress, improve mood, exercise, and have fun—all in one!

E **Evening primrose or starflower oils.** These help reduce breast tenderness, hot flashes, irritability, poor sleep, and vaginal dryness, especially in perimenopause.

F **Friends.** Studies show that meaningful social connection reduces depression and improves positivity. Get through this together with your people!

G **Ghee.** Nothing like a bit of clarified butter for vaginal lubrication.

H **HRT.** Hormone replacement therapy replaces depleted female hormones like estrogen and progesterone, alleviating symptoms of menopause.

I **Iron.** It is important to keep iron levels up when experiencing heavy blood loss to alleviate fatigue, low energy, thinning hair, and brittle nails.

J **Joy. Jokes. Joining.** Find people and things that make you smile and feel alive and connected to help you see beyond the blah times.

K **Kegel exercises.** Strengthening your pelvic floor helps with bladder control and reduces incontinence, as well as relaxing vaginal muscles and aiding vaginal circulation, which helps with lubrication and arousal. So get squeezing!

L Licorice. (Not the candy, but the capsules and root extracts, sorry.) Eating licorice root can reduce the frequency and severity of hot flashes, and licorice in vaginal cream reduces dryness.

M Magnesium. This mineral helps regulate moods, improves sleep quality, and boosts bone mineral density.

N Nourishing food. Fill your plate with healthy fats, fruits and vegetables, whole grains, and quality proteins instead of processed food.

O Oily fish. These are rich in vitamin D, which strengthens bones, and can help combat menopausal depression.

P Probiotic supplements. These help balance the bacteria levels in your body, and studies suggest they can make a positive impact on hot flashes, sleep, mood, weight loss, vaginal dryness, and bone health.

Q Quit smoking. Smoking intensifies menopausal symptoms and can bring them on sooner.

R Red clover. This plant contains natural estrogens, which some studies have shown to relieve hot flashes.

S Soy. It is suggested that a regular soy intake can lower hot flash frequency and severity by 25 percent.

T Turmeric. This spice can help alleviate joint pain, boost heart health, and reduce depression.

U Unwind. Take a bath, spend time in nature, read a great book. Build moments into each day for your body and mind to relax and reset.

V Vaginal creams, lubricants, and gels. There are a range of products that can help vaginal dryness.

W Water. Drink lots of it to maintain hormone levels, prevent muscle cramps, and reduce bloating.

X Exercise. Regular exercise, such as walking, running, or dancing, has been shown to improve sleep, reduce hot flashes, improve mood, and strengthen bones.

Y Yoga. Strengthen muscles and joints, focus your mind, and relax. Yoga can alleviate hot flashes and night sweats, as well as improve mental and physical well-being.

Z Zen. Aim for a Zen state of mind—relax and don't worry about things you can't change. What brings you peace? Put more of that in your life.

YOUR SUPERHEROINE NAME

Is it a bird? Is it a plane? No, it's Captain "Over-These-Ovaries" and their trusty sidekick, you! Use the chart below to find your superheroine name and fill in the blanks:

_____, the _____, _____ of _____
(your name)   (birth month answer)   (partner/friend's   (last trip month answer)
                                                   birth month answer)

	Your birth month	Your partner/friend's birth month	Month you last went on a trip
JAN	Moody	Forgetter	Sanitary Pads
FEB	Itchy	Destroyer	Hot Flashes
MAR	Sweaty	Unleasher	Migraines
APR	Hot	Overthinker	Weight Gain
MAY	Frigid	Avoider	Droopy Boobs
JUN	Snappy	Resister	Libido
JUL	Bloated	Conqueror	Facial Hair
AUG	Hirsute	Crusher	Periods
SEP	Crampy	Delayer	Mood Swings
OCT	Nauseous	Googler	Insomnia
NOV	Dry	Hacker	Anxiety
DEC	Dizzy	Vanquisher	Incontinence

COLOR IN CAPTAIN OVER-THESE-OVARIES
AND DRAW IN YOUR SUPERHEROINE SELF!

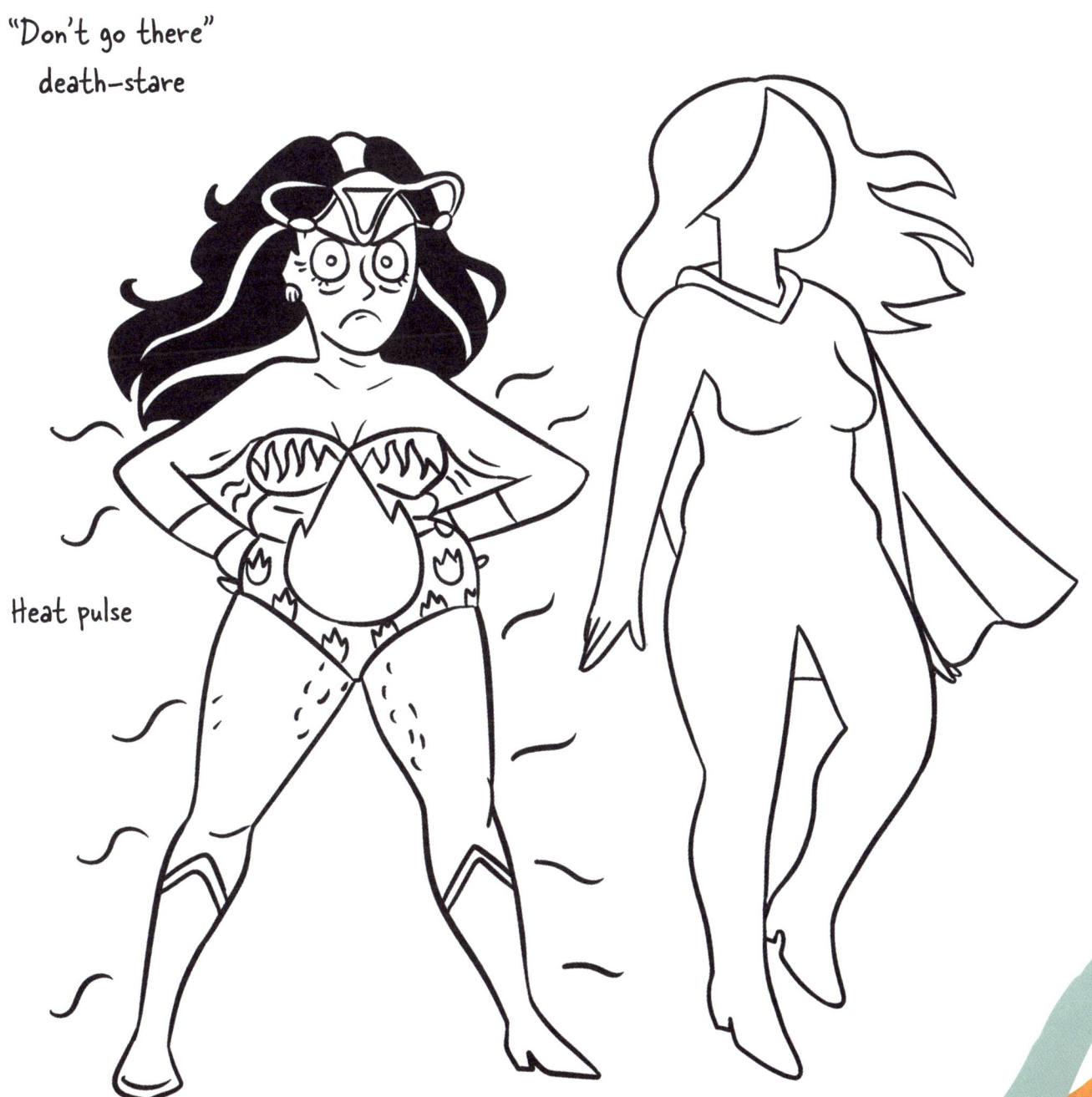

"Don't go there"
death-stare

Heat pulse

I AM AMAZING!

It's easy to knock ourselves and make light of who we are, especially at times like this, when our bodies seem to be in permanent protest. But don't lose sight of reality—YOU are a gift to the world. Of these fifty affirmations, choose *at least* ten that you know are true for you. Hell, choose them all if you want to! You might want to write them up somewhere to remind yourself of who you really are, even when things are a mess.

ACCOMPLISHED	DRIVEN	HUMBLE	RADIANT
AUTHENTIC	EXPERIENCED	INDEPENDENT	REFLECTIVE
BLESSED	FEARLESS	INSPIRATIONAL	SEXY
BOLD	FEISTY	INTELLIGENT	SMART
BRAVE	FIERCE	KIND	SPIRITED
CLASSY	FREE	LOVING	STRONG
CLEVER	FUNNY	MOTIVATED	SUCCESSFUL
COMPASSIONATE	GENEROUS	PASSIONATE	TOUGH
CONFIDENT	GRACEFUL	PERCEPTIVE	TRUTHFUL
COURAGEOUS	GRATEFUL	POSITIVE	UNSTOPPABLE
CREATIVE	HAPPY	POWERFUL	VALUABLE
DEDICATED	HILARIOUS	PROTECTIVE	WISE
	HONEST		WORTHY

```
U N S T O P P A B L E G D E D I C A T E D B H
I N S P I R A T I O N A L N A L O V I N G U I
N A P F N A C C O M P L I S H E D S X Z F G T
T U E C D F G M R K A K N T X F G H Q V I C R
E T R O E U V C O U R A G E O U S I S P E O A
L H C N P Z B T R T S B K R N N U L C V R M D
L E E F E C C G K E I G S J F N J A A K C P I
I N P I N L E Q P R A V E A N Y Q R U I E A A
G T T D D E K X W Y Y T A J T W B I T P O S N
E I I E E V L G P L Y J I T S I E O Q O R S T
N C V N N E U P O E R J T V E E P U G W E I F
T N E T T R A W C B R E V R E D F S R E A O E
S Q D E A H V O G S S I F A U B F I A R P N I
P R O T E C T I V E B Y E L L T G A C F T A S
I H D K F P E L M X N L P N E U H E E U W T T
R O Q N X A U E Y Y F E E P C C A F F L O E Y
I N K J J F A S Y Y E N R S O E T B U M R S W
T E S F E E S E V R A J R O S S D I L L T T I
E S F T L A B R F O R N L A U E I P V E H R S
D T A B L V H O Z G L N F J Y S D T L E Y O E
V R M C Q V M B L R E V H I Q Y D R I V E N C
G U Y B K T M S O D S M A R T N S B Y V K G G
H L C C T O U G H K S U C C E S S F U L E D O
```

Answers on page 93.

THE MENOPAUSAL ROLLER COASTER

Menopause isn't all bad. There are highs and lows, and some things throw you for a loop. What are yours? Write in the joys and frustrations of your own roller-coaster ride.

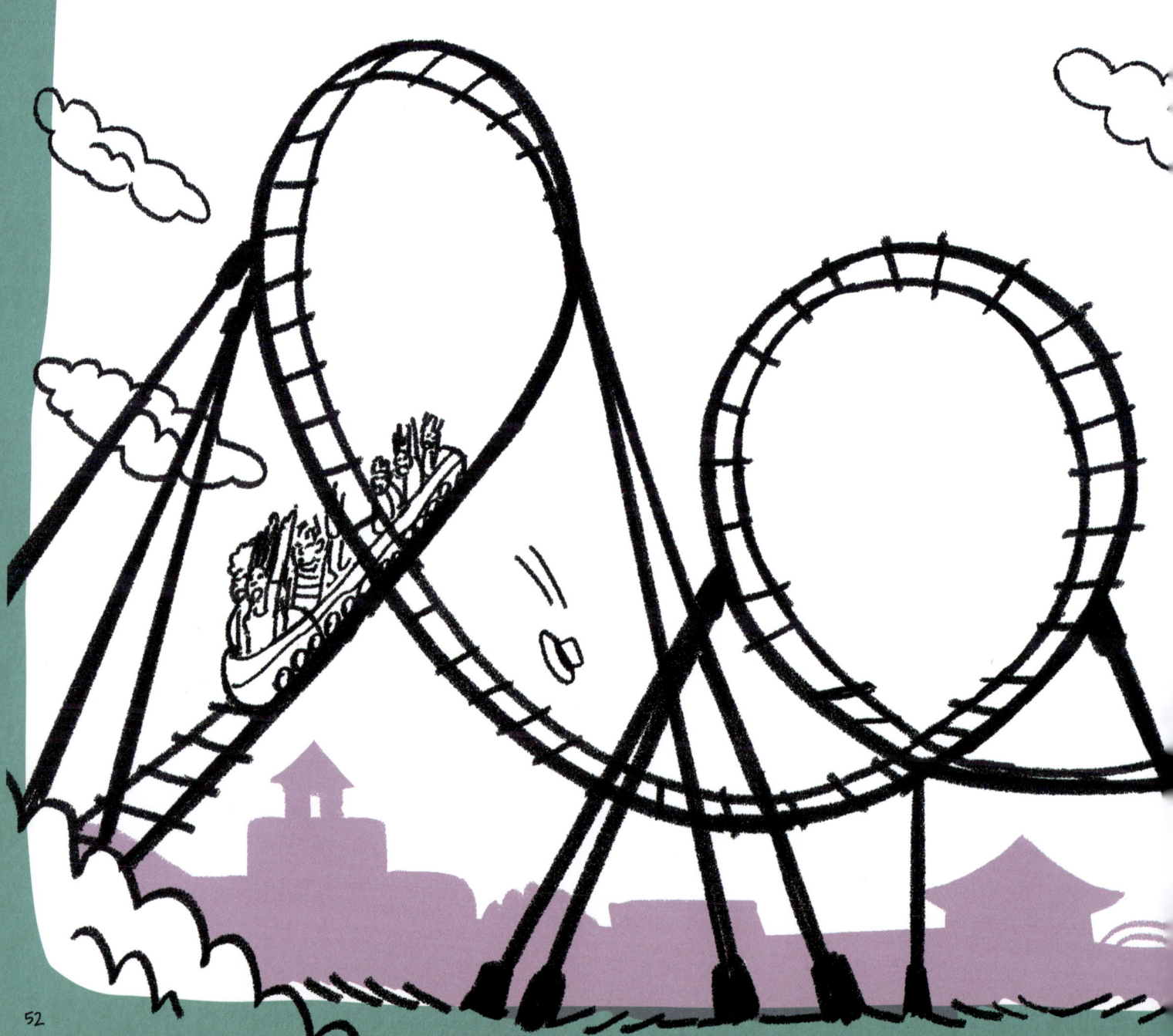

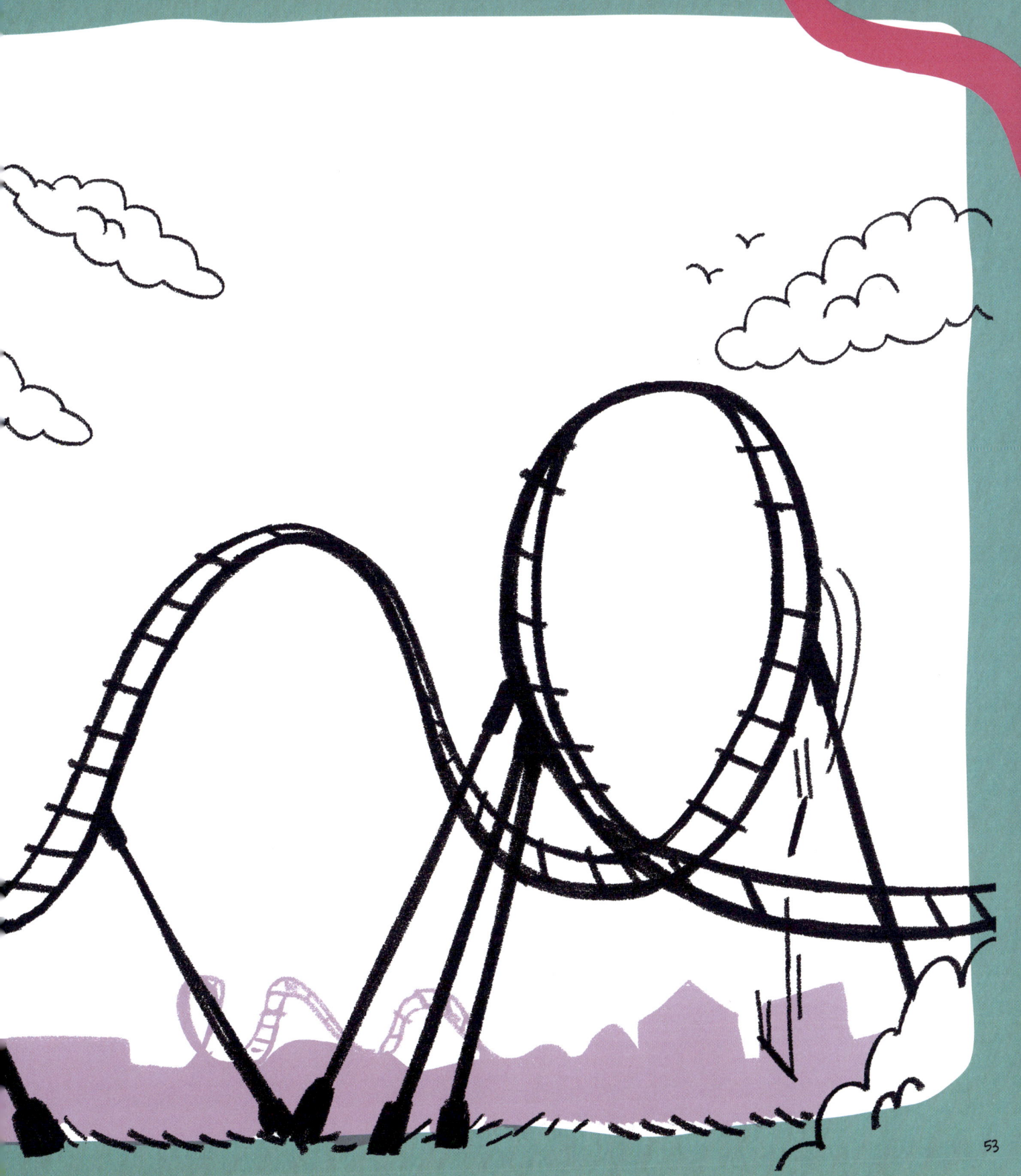

SYMPTOM SCRAMBLE

Unscramble these symptoms that some people get with perimenopause. Don't worry, you won't necessarily experience all of these. Or at least not all at once!

LISAHOTSI _____

EAAUSN _____

EATUGIF _____

EIISNCSHT _____

MNINAISO _____

NNSIIUTT _____

IOSTNPCTAINO _____

PSSSTEOIOOOR _____

EDHASHACE _____

XIEAYNT _____

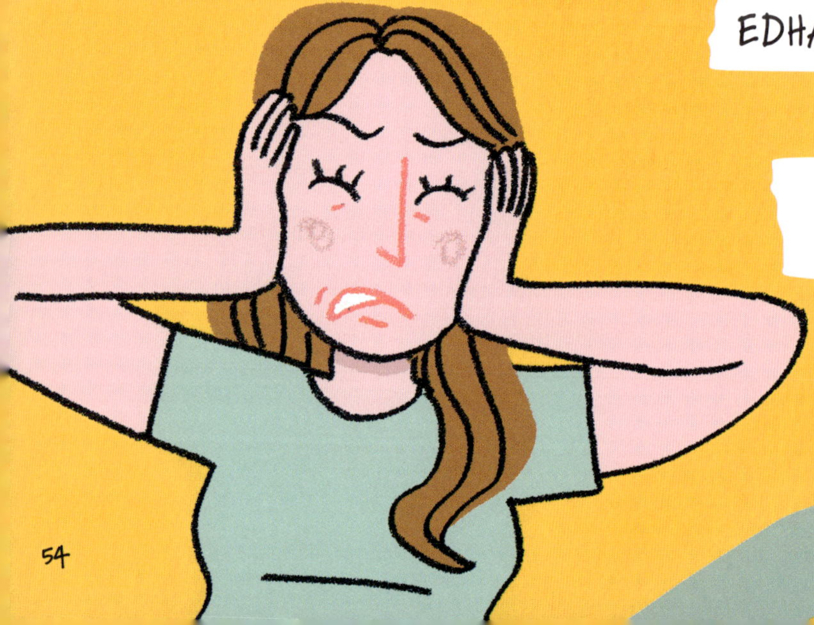

Answers on page 94.

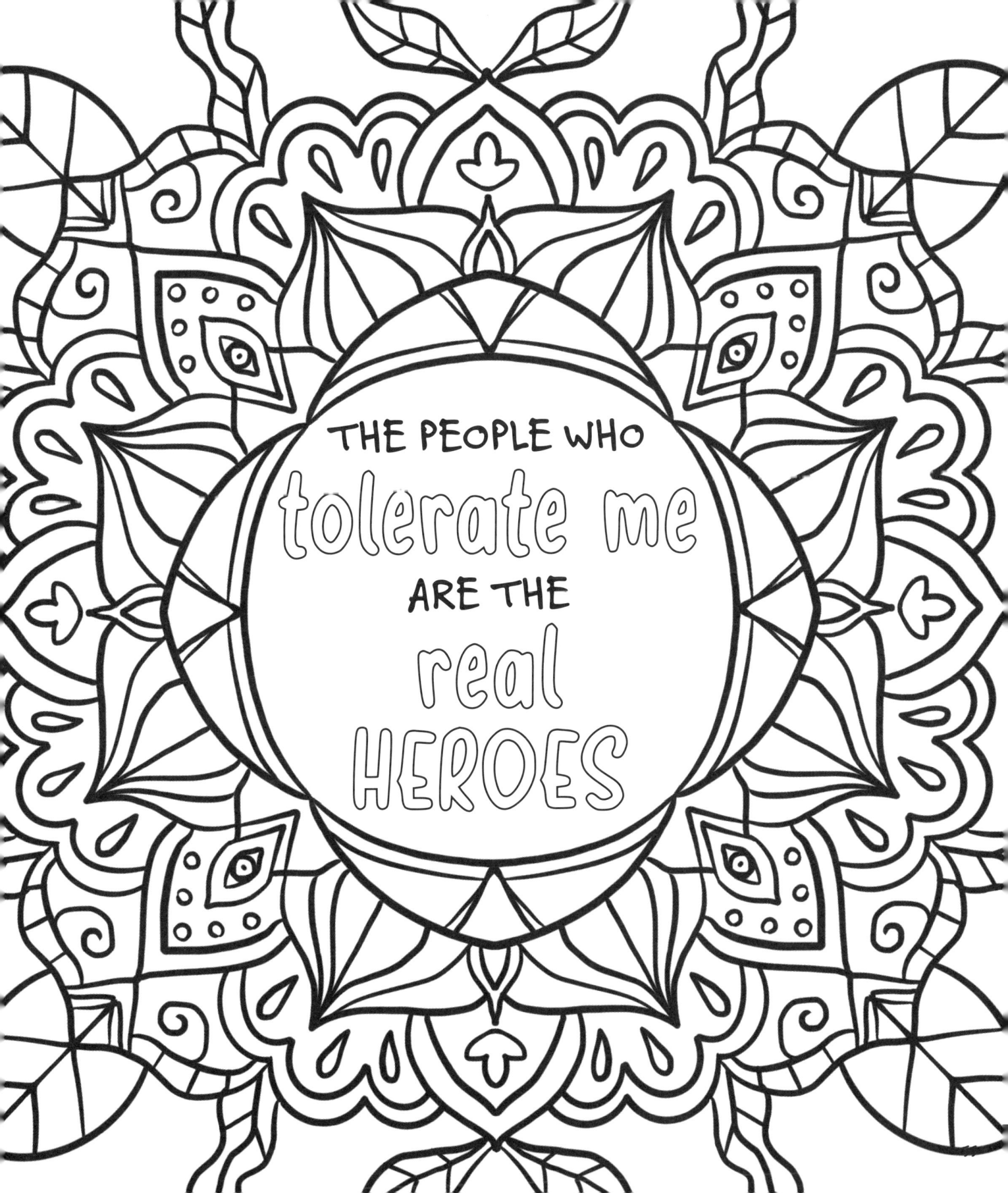

JUST A TYPICAL DAY

Maybe this isn't a typical day in your life, or maybe it is? If you have a friend nearby, hand them this page so they can write your answers in or do it yourself while trying not to peek at the story.

The alarm clock rang, shocking me awake. I'd only managed to drop off a few

hours earlier. Not enough sleep—again! I'd spent most of the night

_____ —again.
(something you do before you fall asleep)

Shuffling to the mirror, it seemed a(n) _____ was looking
                                        (animal)

back at me, with hideous_____ and fang—like _____.
                        (facial feature)   (another facial feature)

Slugging back my morning _____, I had to hurry now, or I would be
                         (alcoholic drink)

late for the _____.
             (black-tie event)

Now, where's my _____? I looked under the_____.
                (essential item you need for going out)   (furniture)

Nope. The _____, in the _____, even the
          (room in your home)   (where you keep valuables)

_____. Just gone. What was I going to do?
(part of your home you go to the least)

Slumping down on the couch, I decided I couldn't go out that day, so I

_____ and _____ instead. This continued for
(what you do to get comfortable)   (something you enjoy doing)

_____ until I got hungry and went to get some _____
(period of time)   (snack)

from the kitchen. There, sitting smugly, was my _____.
                                                 (same essential item)

Too bad, I didn't feel like going out anymore, and more importantly,

_____?
(something you're wondering about at the moment)

YOUR MENOPAUSAL SPIRIT ANIMAL

Looking at the illustrations, which of these animals speaks to you? Let them be your perimenopausal guide and find out which characteristics you may already embody or may come to embody with their help! Stick their pictures on the fridge, tattoo them on your arm, and let their wonderful examples carry you through the rougher times!

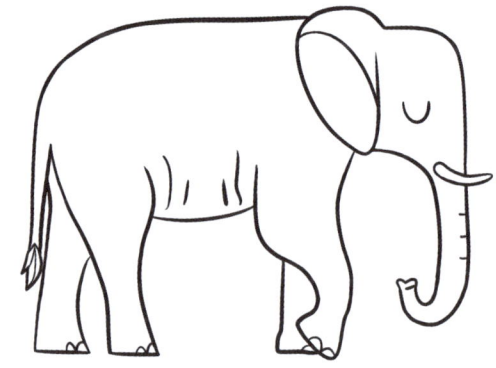

Elephant: They carry a little more around the hips than they might like, but these creatures don't let anything weigh them down. They can choose to be gentle or crash onto a scene and are anything but invisible. Social bonds are important, and they support and nurture each other, sticking together through thick and thin. Elephant herds are matriarchal—the oldest, most dominant females hold their families together, providing stability and guidance. Damn straight they do! Commanding, confident, supportive, and wise, just like you!

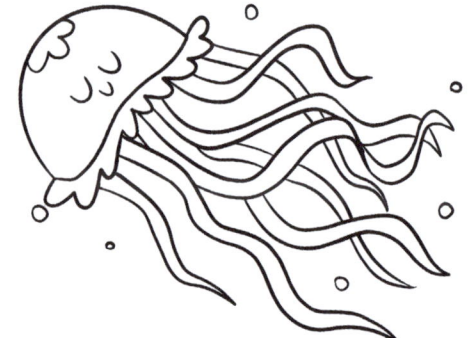

Jellyfish: Sure, they're wobbly and bag-like, but jellyfish are also graceful, riding the currents wherever they are taken. Their barbed tentacles make them unforgettable to any who cross them the wrong way. In the depths of the ocean, some are also bioluminescent, glowing as they float. Jellyfish have been around since before the dinosaurs, so they're doing something right. They're made of 95 percent water and are a bit floppy, yes, but you are gorgeous and dangerous, jelly queen.

Dolphin: Leaping and surfing with obvious joy and a sense of playfulness, dolphins turn obstacles into adventures, riding wave after wave. Known for their strong social bonds, dolphins help each other with hunting, raising young, and even lifting sick ones to the ocean's surface to breathe when things get too much for them. Despite their mammal roots, dolphins don't have hair, but they still look cute, so don't sweat the hair loss, sis!

Cat: With nine lives and the uncanny ability to land on their feet, cats epitomize a nonchalant, "no more f#@ks to give" approach to life. They are independent, great at self-care, demand what they want (even if it is at 3 a.m.), and seek affection on their own terms. They take time to trust people, but once that has been earned, they are a friend for life. Swaying, swaggering, swishing, purring, hissing, or swiping, they go where and when they want and let you know exactly how they feel. You are the embodiment of confidence.

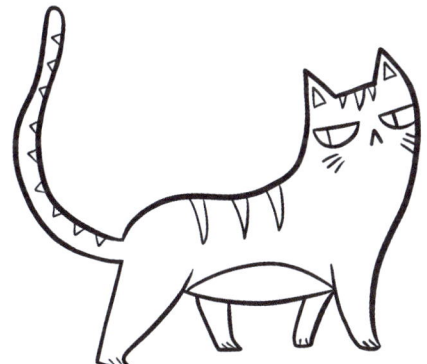

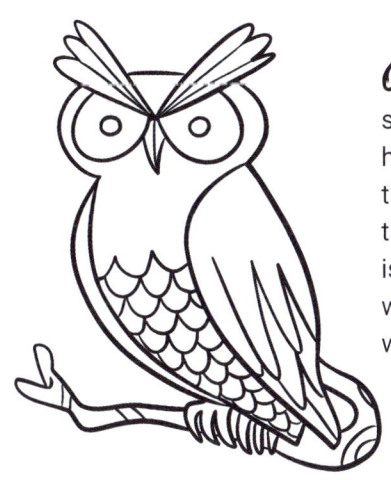

Owl: Watchful and wise, owls navigate the dark and unknown with ease, seeking opportunities when others might just see inky blackness. They have flexible necks, so they can easily turn to see what's going on, and their powerful ears zero in on the slightest sound. They don't advertise themselves—their feathers silence their flight. But what isn't said in words is shown in action—these birds mean business. In Greek mythology, the owl was connected with Athena, goddess of war. The owl tackles challenges with wisdom, quietly getting on with it when others might back off, just like you.

Flamingo: Vibrant and gorgeous, with long legs and plumage to die for, these birds exude grace and poise and are experts at the balancing act, standing on one leg for hours. Do you know what a group of flamingos is called? A flamboyance! Yas, queen! That has you and your friends written all over it! Ravishing, balanced, social, and persistent—what more could you want?

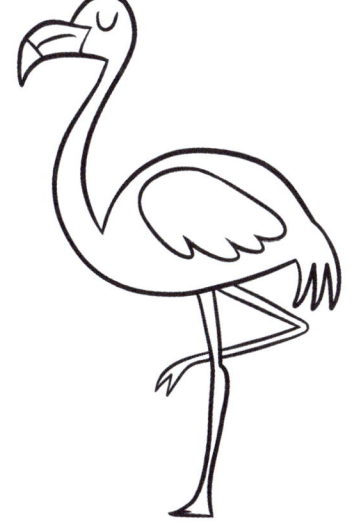

A HOT FLASH-BACK THROUGH HISTORY

Test your knowledge about menopause around the world and through history.

1. **The term *menopause* was created in this year. Too bad for you if you lived before then!**

    a. 1637   b. 1749   c. 1821   d. 1915

2. **Match these delightful translations for menopause with the correct languages.**

Month of Stopping	Japanese
Second Spring	Greek
Years of Renewing Energy	Arabic
The Hopeless Age	Chinese

3. **Horse pee, anyone? Urine from pregnant horses was harvested to "treat" menopause during which time period?**

    a. 1790s   b. 1850s   c. 1920s   d. 1940s

4. **Let's learn from the Japanese! Hot flashes tend to be less common there. It has been suggested that this is due to:**

    a. Frequent hot baths

    b. Higher natural body temperature in Japanese people

    c. High soy intake

    d. Much more active lifestyle

5. **In historic times, you might have been given the following to eat to help with menopausal symptoms (lucky you!):**

    a. Crushed cow ovaries and juiced testicles

    b. Goat placentas boiled in colostrum

    c. Ground deer antlers

    d. All of the above

6. **If you're from one of these ethnic groups, sorry to tell you, but research suggests that menopause starts earlier in life for you:**

   a. Southeast Asian or Arabic

   b. Caucasian or Chinese

   c. Black or Hispanic

   d. Pacific Islander or Indigenous peoples of the Americas

7. **Be glad you didn't have menopause during Victorian times! You could have faced the following to "help" you:**

   a. Been diagnosed with "climacteric insanity" and locked in an asylum

   b. Had your ovaries removed to make you more docile and hardworking

   c. Had your clitoris removed to stop your hysteria, idiocy, or mania

   d. All of the above

8. **If you were an ancient Greek, you might have believed that menopausal symptoms were because:**

   a. Your uterus moved around your body

   b. There was a blockage of flow of your "essential wind," especially in the neck

   c. Your menstrual blood was putrefied and turned to poison

   d. You exhibited bad behavior in your youth

9. **In 1966, Dr. Robert Wilson wrote a book called *Feminine Forever*. In it, he calls menopause a:**

   a. Dried spring

   b. Descending hell

   c. Galloping catastrophe

   d. Wilted flower

10. **Pliny the Elder, the Roman philosopher, believed that menstruating women could:**

    a. Turn wine into water

    b. Kill bees

    c. Make crops grow faster

    d. Shatter mirrors

Answers on page 94.

FORTY SYMPTOMS FOR THE OVER-FORTY CROWD

How many symptoms of menopause are there? Only you know for you! Find as many of our top forty as you can in this word find. Circle any you've experienced.

ABDOMINAL FAT

ACHES

ANXIETY

BAD PMS

BONE DENSITY LOSS

BRAIN FOG

BURNING TONGUE

DEPRESSION

DIZZINESS

DRY MOUTH

DRY SKIN

FACIAL HAIR

FATIGUE

HEADACHES

HEAVY OR LIGHT PERIODS

HOT FLASHES

INSOMNIA

INTERRUPTED SLEEP

IRREGULAR PERIODS

IRRITABILITY

ITCHINESS

JOINT PAIN

LOW LIBIDO

MEMORY LOSS

MIGRAINES

MOOD SWINGS

MUSCLE LOSS

MUSCLE PAIN

NAUSEA

NIGHT SWEATS

PERIOD PAIN

PINS AND NEEDLES

POOR FOCUS

TENSE MUSCLES

THINNING HAIR

UNMOTIVATED

UTIs

VAGINAL DRYNESS

WEAK BLADDER

WEIGHT GAIN

```
H M W E A K B L A D D E R T H I N N I N G H A I R
E E E Z L N F M O W W S X T U J K V O B E B U N N
A M I S U T S L W D M T O W K N Y I R E F U I T X
V O G M U S C L E P A I N K C P S R N M R R R E S
Y R H H J R E J D M J V N L R S G R Q Y Q N R R B
O Y T C Z Z A L R S I I F E P T I T R X I E R U
R L G P P O B H M J Y U N R B Z B T H S B N G U I
L O A I C J M G Y X X M P S J B R A V K O G U P S
I S I N H H H F F T Y E O J O U A B A C N T L T H
G S N S M F T F A T D M N U G M I I G Z E O A E N
H A B A U D P B E C Z W M S T U N L I O D N R D H
T D B N W Q D I Z Z I N E S S H F I N U E G P S E
P W D D F B X J W L F A J N S Q O T A N N U E L A
E C K N O N F X O J O R L S G H G Y L A S E R E D
R J K E A M H S F I F W E H U Z F L D U I I I E A
I M O E A M I F F C N N L W A T L E R S T H O P C
O I K D O O Q N O V I T W I P I U E Y E Y O D E H
D G P L O O I J A H T A P Q B G R T N A L T S R E
S R E E Q D V O C L D Y B A I I T N E D O F D I S
V A U S G S D T K J F D I T I D D P S C S L R O D
X I X D K W I A U N I A A J Y N Z O S A S A Y D H
U N M O T I V A T E D F T P O O R F O C U S S P I
U E D Z Q N A N I G H T S W E A T S C H X H K A T
I S R B Q G M U S C L E L O S S M W V E P E I I B
I J T E N S E M U S C L E S S K H I V S J S N N M
```

Answers on page 94.

WHAT FILLS YOUR BUCKET?

When your bucket is full, you feel confident, calm, patient, secure, friendly, and positive. Sometimes it can fill to overflowing and spreads to others. What are you grateful for right now? Fill your bucket with as many things as you can think of, drawn or written, and never mind about that unfortunate horse pee bucket image from page 60.

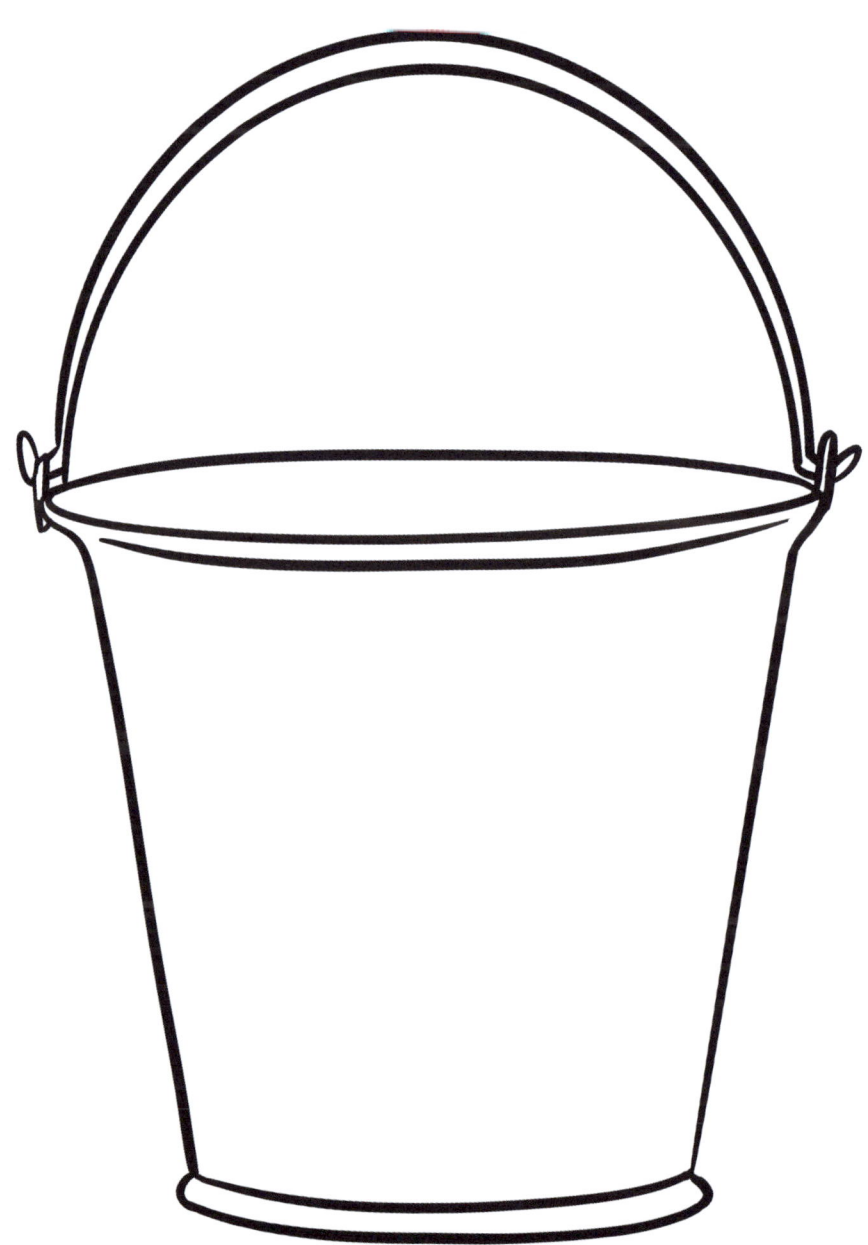

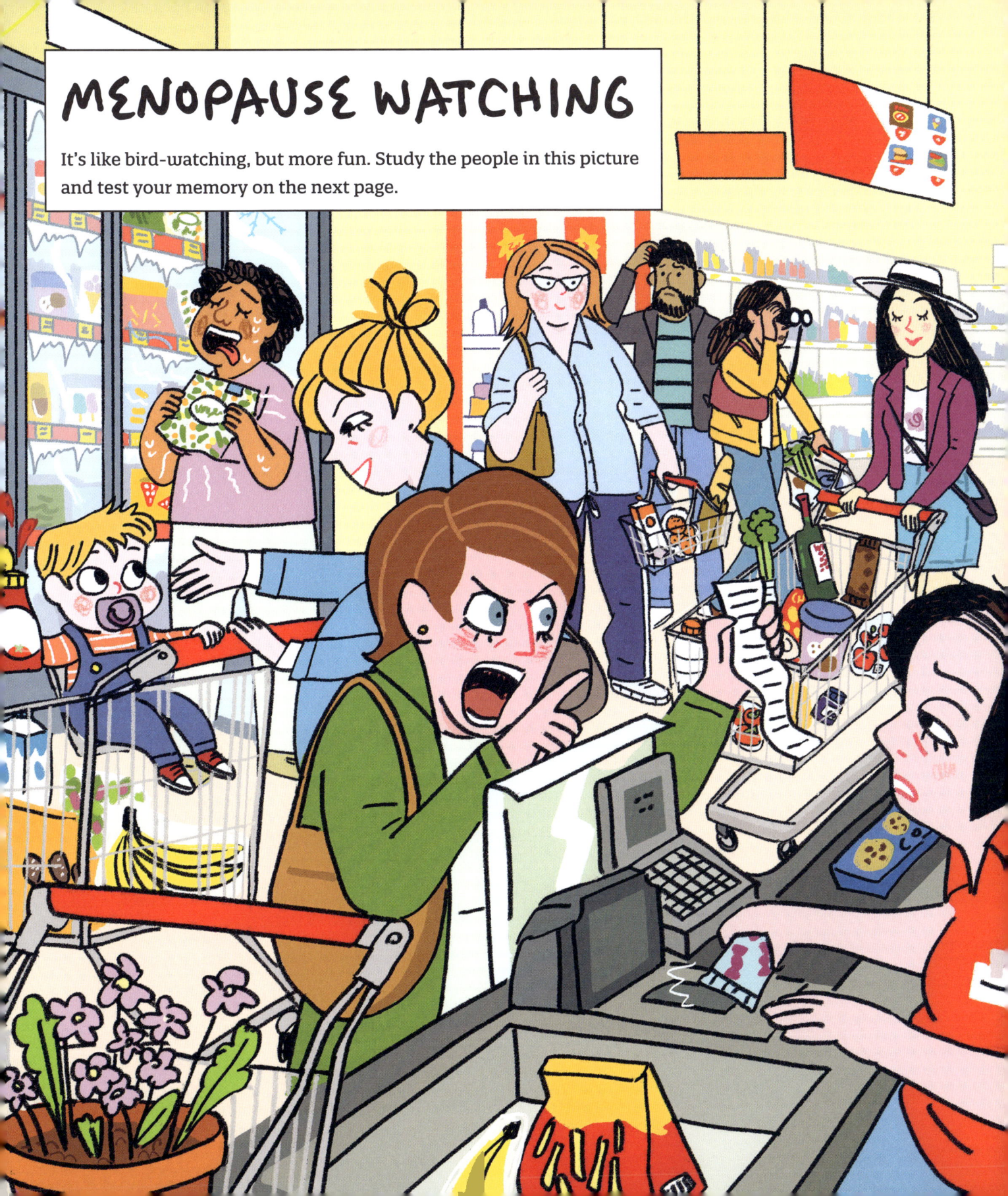

Can you remember what you saw in the picture on the last page? Try answering these questions about it. Did you need to peek?

1. How many shopping carts did you see? _____

2. How many shopping baskets did you see? _____

3. What was in the shopping cart with the upset customer? _____

4. How did one customer deal with their hot flash? _____

5. Who looked exhausted? _____

6. What was the baby holding? _____

7. What was the checkout operator scanning? _____

8. What signs of menopause did you notice in the picture? _____

Answers on page 94.

MONALISA TOUCH

I swear I am not making this up: the MonaLisa Touch® treatment uses lasers to make tiny cuts in your vaginal wall, stimulating the regrowth of blood vessels, collagen, and elastin. How crazy is that? Apparently, it can help treat dryness, itchiness, and painful sex. It takes five minutes, and the best bit, they say it doesn't hurt! This is all I will be able to picture, though, if I go through with it.

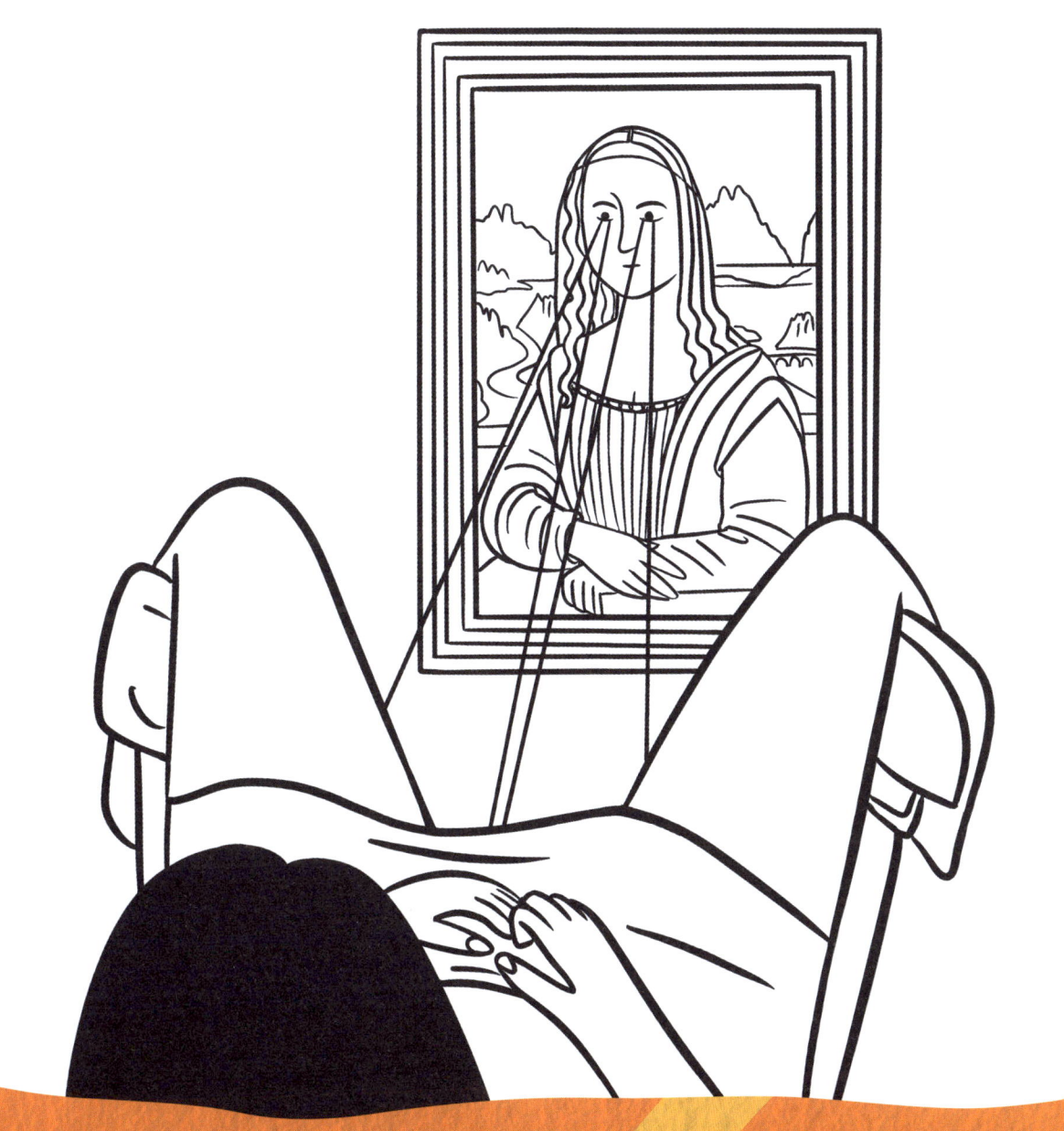

TALES OF TRANSFORMATION

What kind of monster has menopause turned you into? The full moon turns some into werewolves, and it seems that menopause can bring out our scary alter egos, too! Answer the following questions honestly to find out!

1. **I am most likely to keep this close to me at all times:**
   a. My pillow
   b. A fan
   c. Chocolate!
   d. Aspirin
   e. My keys, so I don't lose them again
   f. My hand. Talk to it.

2. **The worst things to say to me during menopause:**
   a. You look like you haven't slept in days.
   b. It's freezing in here. I'm going to close the window.
   c. You might want to cut back on those desserts—you're getting a bit of a tummy there!
   d. Come on, you're fine. Get over it.
   e. I didn't make the reservation. YOU made the reservation!
   f. Just be quiet. That's safest.

3. **You are most likely to find me:**
   a. Asleep in front of the TV
   b. By an open window or under an A/C unit
   c. Browsing the pantry
   d. In the doctor's waiting room
   e. In the laundry room with a tomato, wondering what the hell I'm doing
   f. Crying, laughing, or flipping out

4. **If I were a piece of playground equipment, I would be:**
   a. A slide
   b. Anything metal that gets superhot in the sun and burns you when you touch it
   c. A trampoline
   d. Broken
   e. A maze
   f. A swing set

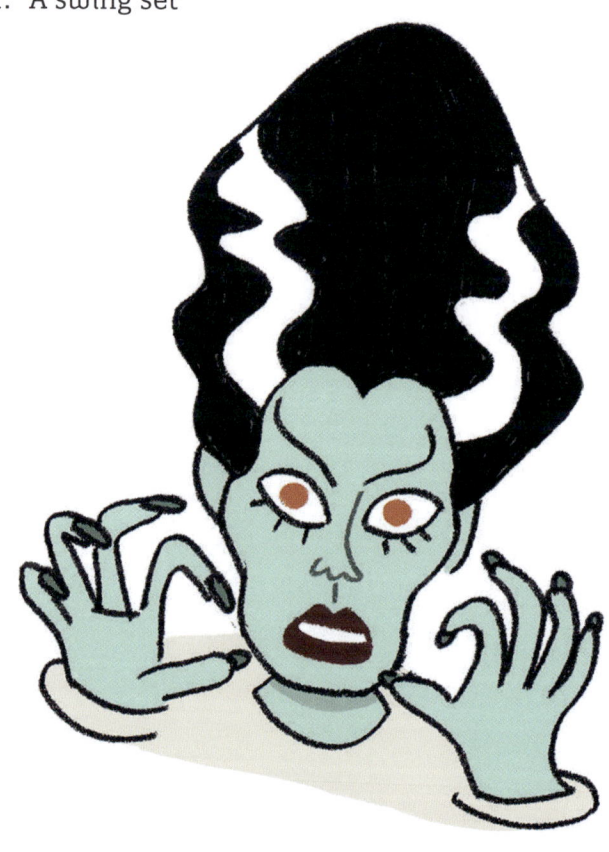

5. **The best song to describe me is:**
   a. "Zombie," by The Cranberries
   b. "Hot Stuff," by Donna Summer
   c. "Fat Bottomed Girls," by Queen
   d. "Super Freak," by Rick James
   e. "What's Going On," by Marvin Gaye
   f. "Maneater," by Hall & Oates

6. **Time for some lovin'. The problem is:**
   a. I'm already asleep.
   b. I'm a sweaty mess before anything happens.
   c. There's no problem. Don't like my hairy legs or tummy? Deal with it!
   d. It's drier than a desert down there. Good luck!
   e. I'd invite you in, but I just can't find my keys.
   f. I just remembered a TV show I saw last week. Now I'm sad. No, I don't know why. Shut up and pass me a tissue. And NO, you're not getting lucky, you creep!

7. **My spirit animal is:**
   a. Sloth
   b. Camel
   c. Panda
   d. Porcupine
   e. Goldfish
   f. Black widow spider

8. **You'll find me drinking:**
   a. Coffee, extra extra strong
   b. Ice cold water, with ice
   c. Hot chocolate, wine, or something sweet
   d. Ural® sachets or cranberry juice
   e. Oh shoot! I put the kettle on three hours ago!
   f. The tears of all who dare look at me today

9. **My dream vacation would be:**
   a. Lying under a beach umbrella, somewhere peaceful
   b. Antarctica
   c. An all-inclusive cruise
   d. Somewhere I can get a massage
   e. No point. I'll never find my passport.
   f. Staycation, alone

10. **My favorite time of the year is:**
    a. Bedtime
    b. Winter
    c. Every day!
    d. 20 years ago
    e. Hang on—what day is it now?
    f. How the hell should I know?!

11. **The best movie or TV show title to describe me is:**
    a. *Sleepless in Seattle*
    b. *The Flash*
    c. *As Good as It Gets*
    d. *Misery*
    e. *Dude, Where's My Car?*
    f. *10 Things I Hate About You*

Which letter did you answer the most? Turn to page 94 to discover which monster you are most like.

THIS GIRL IS ON FIRE!

Think hot flashes don't have their advantages? Think again! You can now:

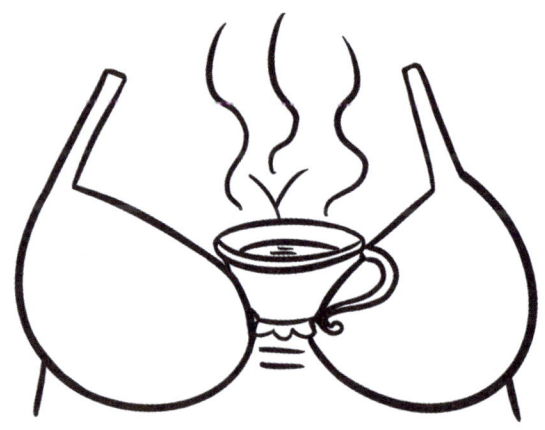

BE A HEAT LAMP FOR
BABY ANIMALS

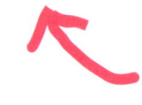

BOIL WATER
FOR DRINKS

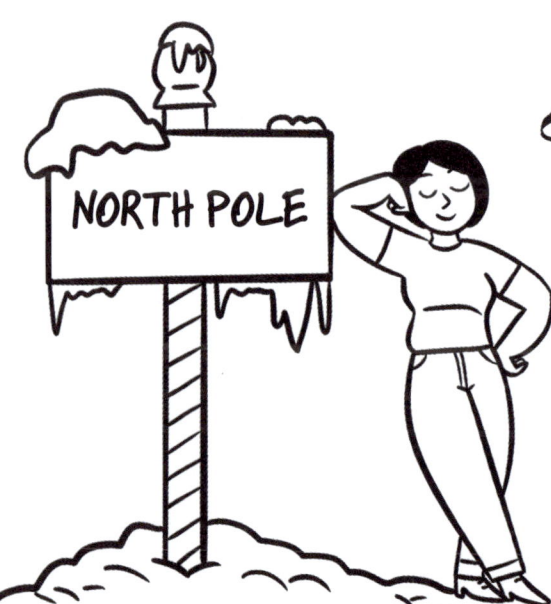

ACCLIMATE EASILY
AT THE POLES

SOMETIMES I FEEL LIKE . . .

It's okay to have days where you feel like a broken-down car. Circle or write in what's making you most unhappy. Take a break to color this in and see how you feel afterward.

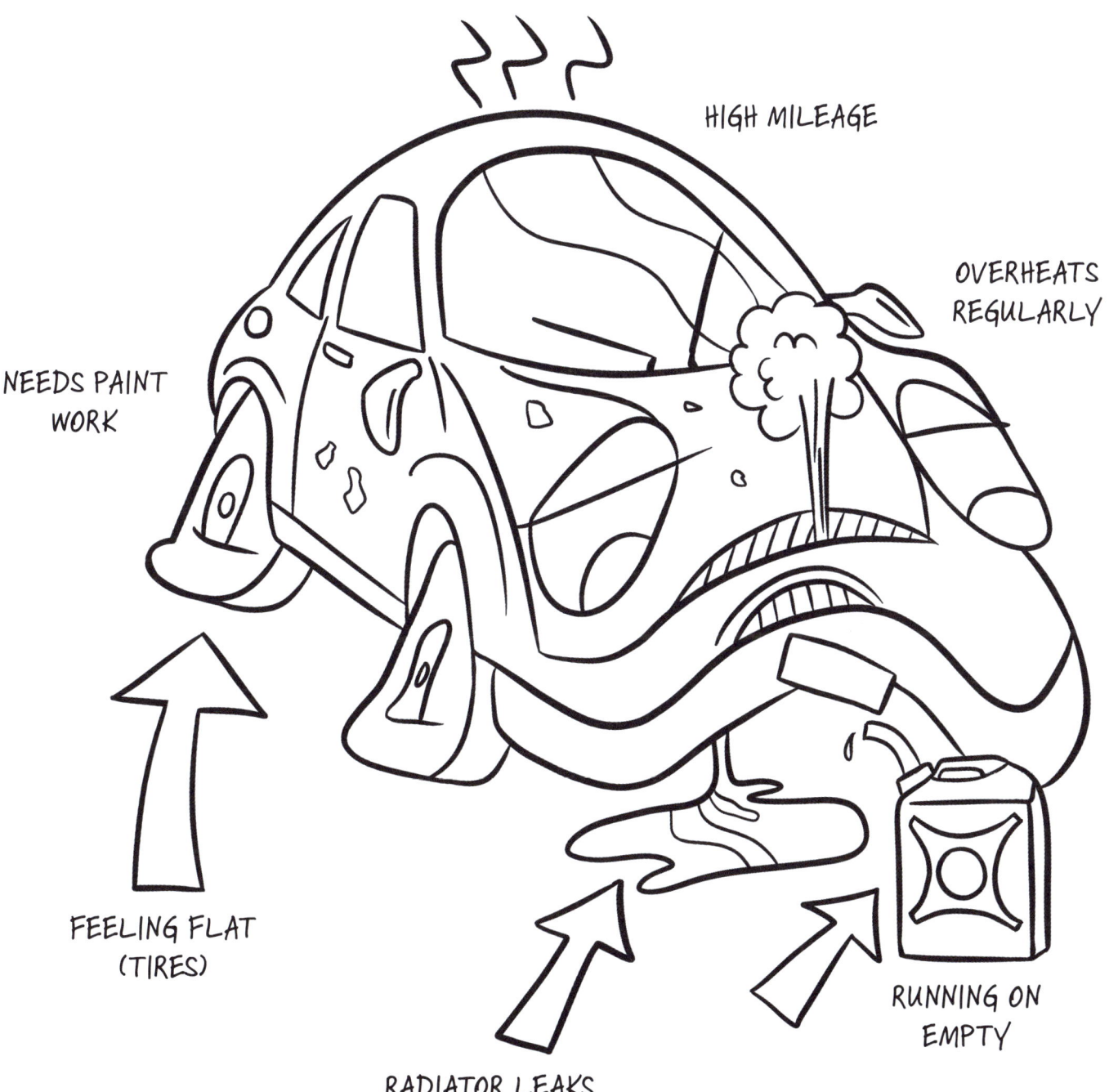

HIGH MILEAGE

OVERHEATS REGULARLY

NEEDS PAINT WORK

FEELING FLAT (TIRES)

RADIATOR LEAKS

RUNNING ON EMPTY

BRA-VOLUTION

Much like photos or popular songs can remind us of the landmarks of our lives, I reckon our bras can too! The humble bra starts off as something so exciting for girls, a step into long anticipated and mysterious "womanhood." Then, confidently and completely impractically, cute and sexy bras show us living life to the fullest as young things, only to be replaced by more sensible ones as responsibilities like work and motherhood make their marks. At some point, we know who we are and don't care what others think anymore. Our bras end up reflecting this too. What a journey our boob-holders can tell!

WHERE ARE YOU ON YOUR BRA-VOLUTION TIMELINE?

A What Are We Training For? Bra
You reached puberty! And to celebrate you probably had an awkward shopping experience for a training bra that everyone noticed the first time you wore a white shirt.

B More Padded Than a Lock-Up Cell Bra
Wow, chica—check out your shape! Yes, we all know there's more padding than breasts in your bra, but fake it till we make it, am I right?

C Squee Bra
So cute! Look at the colors! The polka dots! The frills! This bra is sexy but not mature. It must withstand hikes up hills, dancing in clubs, careless washes with other colors, the possibility of being seen. It screams, "I am young! I am fun! The world is all mine!"

D Brafessional
You've got to look the part at work, so cute apple prints and frills poking through on your straps won't cut it anymore. So bring on the satin, plain colors, and underwire, and get to work!

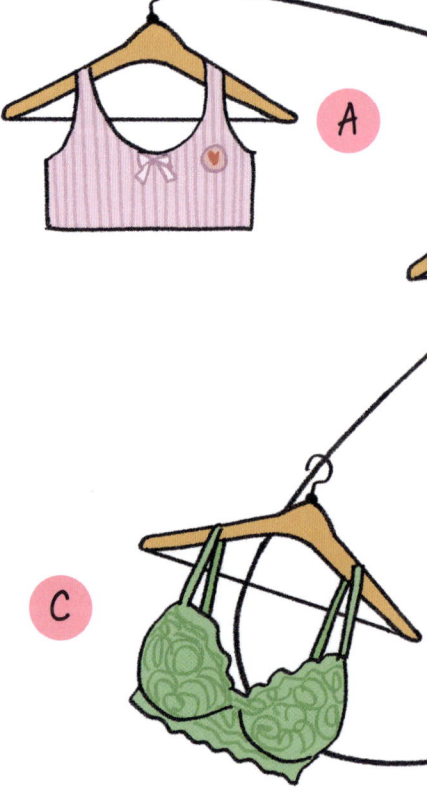

E Barely There Bra

You pair this sexy but ultimately useless number with a matching thong, wear them for a few minutes, and then they spend the rest of the night on the floor.

F Mama Bra

Too much Barely There Bra time might lead to this one. Designed for breasts that expand exponentially and complete with peekaboo flaps for baby to reach their favorite assets.

G Milker Bra

You feel like a cow but hey, you are a mother goddess who is making milk for her baby, so it's still a win. And at least you can text hands-free with this number on.

H Sensible Bra

You've got far too much to do these days, and itchy or squeezy bras just don't cut it anymore. You opt for a wider band, strong shoulders, and good support without feeling like you're being chopped and chaffed under your shirts.

I No Bra

As free as the wind blows. What's the point? Be free, you lioness!

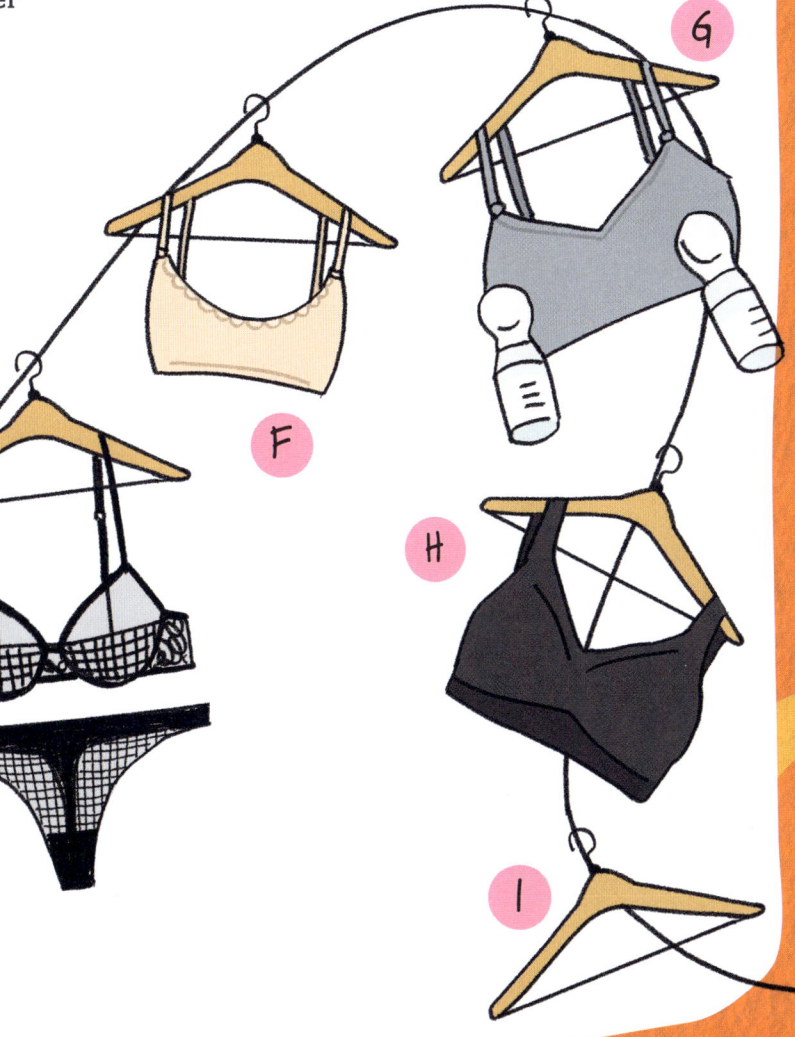

MAKE IT AN EVENT!

Menopause can feel like a time of loss, like a letting go of youth, beauty, and vitality. Perhaps the best way to see this phase as the healthy, normal part of life that it is is to commemorate and even celebrate it. In our culture, there are no ceremonies to mark the onset or fulfillment of menopause, so let's do something special and affirming for ourselves! Can we not make time for a "Hurray, well done, you get to rest those ovaries now"? And why settle for just one event? Perimenopause is a transition—let's prepare ourselves and acknowledge it. Menopause is the finish line—so mark the occasion with those you love!

Use this handy planner for both events and let's make some new traditions!

PLANNING

Choose any of these suggestions below and add your own ideas for the opposite of a pity party, but a celebration of this stage of your life!

THEME

- ☐ **Comfort:** No heels or uncomfortable clothing allowed!

- ☐ **Hot stuff:** Dress to impress or to survive a sudden hot flash. Have a firepit or lots of candles, or really splash out and go somewhere tropical together—or to a sauna!

- ☐ **Puberty era:** What decade was it when you got your first period? Now that you're getting your last, relive those fashionable moments in music, dress, and decor.

- ☐ **Pajama party:** Why not make it a sleepover and wear your favorite pj's?

- ☐ **Paint the town red:** We are, after all, farewelling Aunt Flo, so you may as well decorate and wear the color!

ADD YOUR IDEAS HERE:

_____

FOOD AND DRINK

- ☐ **Comfort food:** Chocolate, wine, sinful treats, cocktails. Or how about an ovary-shaped cake or cupcakes with red centers?

- ☐ **Healthy delights:** Is this a new phase of health awareness? Showcase it with fruit platters or smoothies.

- ☐ **Bloody Marys:** Need I say more?

- ☐ **Make it red:** Raspberries, strawberries, cherries, ketchup, watermelon, tomato soup— you get the idea!

ADD YOUR IDEAS HERE:

_____

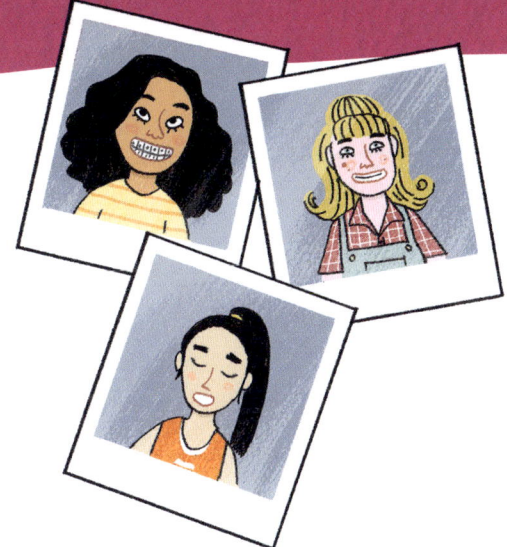

ENTERTAINMENT

☐ **Pampering session:** Either bring in the professionals or do it yourselves. Face masks, manicures, foot spas, etc.

☐ **Match the photos:** Have everyone bring photos of them during puberty. Can you tell who is who?

☐ **Ovary piñata:** Either fill it with treats (red is best) or absolutely nothing! After all, menopause is about the ovaries no longer producing, right? Another thing you could do is gather quotes and encouraging notes from older women, either famous ones or people you value. Fold these up and fill the piñata with them for people to read and share with each other.

☐ **Do something healthy and invigorating together:** Take a yoga or dance class, go on a hike, visit a health or well-being center, kayak, sing karaoke! Feel good about your bodies and what you can do with them.

☐ **Bring in an expert:** Have a chef do a cooking class, take a painting class, or learn a new skill together.

ADD YOUR IDEAS HERE:

_____

CEREMONY

☐ **Letting go ritual:** Write down the things you are saying goodbye to at this stage of life, good and bad. Contemplate each one as you let it go. You could burn them in a fire, write with chalk on rocks to throw into the sea or a lake, or use leaves as symbols and release them into a fast-flowing stream.

☐ **Those who have gone before:** Invite special people who are on the other side of menopause. Give them time to share their stories and answer questions. Then let them surround you to speak words of affirmation or say prayers over you. You may choose to symbolize this time with an exchange of gifts.

☐ **New moon observation:** Go outside and make a bonfire on the night of a new moon. Share with your loved ones about this new phase of life, what you are looking forward to and what you are less sure of. You may even want to dance in the moonlight, howl at the moon, or stay up to see the sunrise.

☐ **Special planting:** Choose something to plant together with your loved ones. As you and they dig away the soil, reflect on what is being removed from your life. Plant the seed or sapling, while reflecting on this unknown time, your hopes for this next phase of life, and how you will support each other.

☐ **Marking the occasion:** Why not commemorate this time with a new piercing or tattoo? Have it done in the company of those special to you and use it as a time to explain its significance to you.

ADD YOUR IDEAS HERE:

_____

MY AMAZING MEMORY

I have a great memory! For example,

my first teacher was _____

my childhood phone number was _____

my first crush was _____

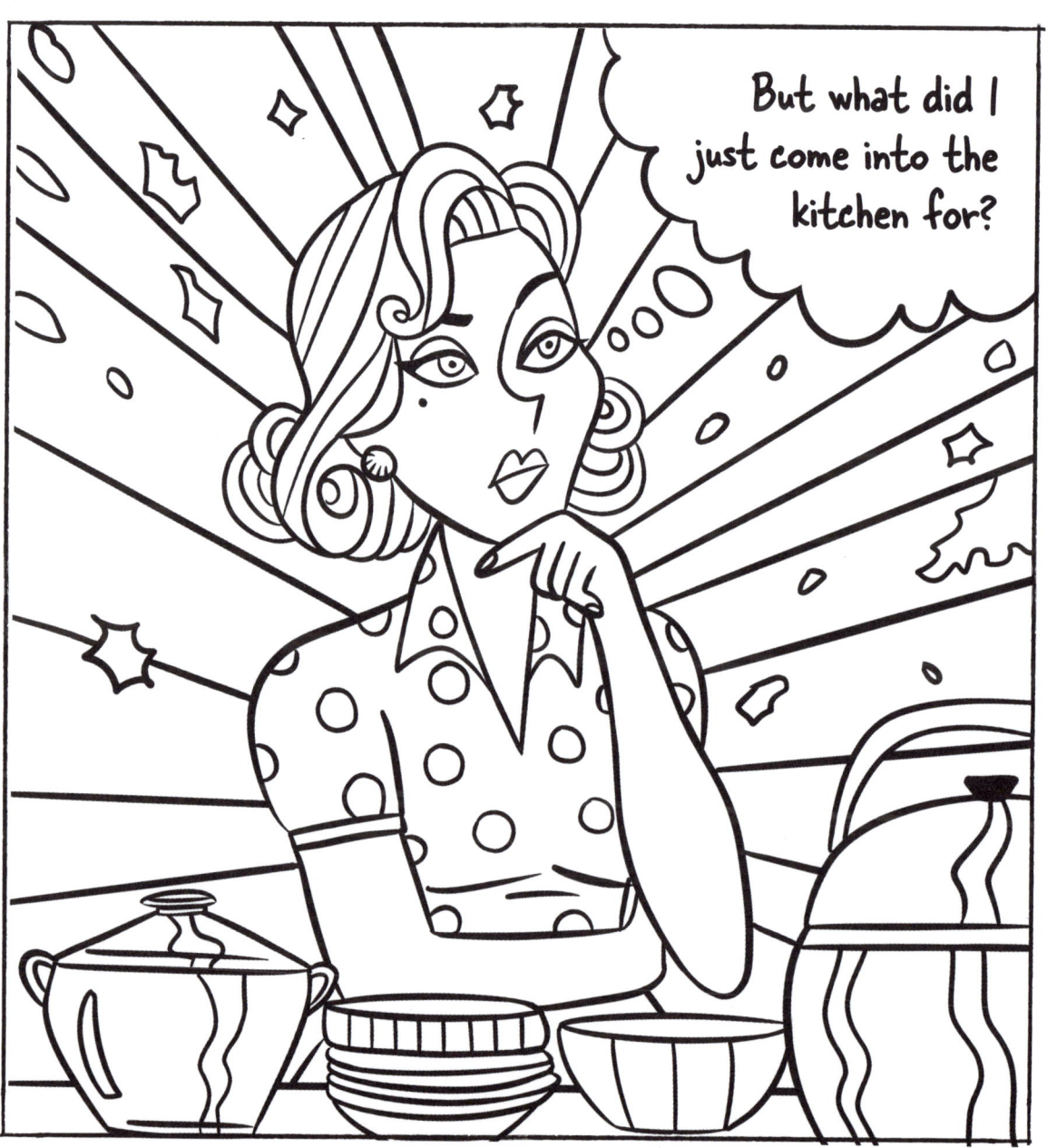

SHOUT! LET IT ALL OUT!

I get it. Sometimes things (or people) are too much and you just need to car-scream. Use this page as a safe venting space. Scribble, swear, write what you'd really like to say. Let it all out!

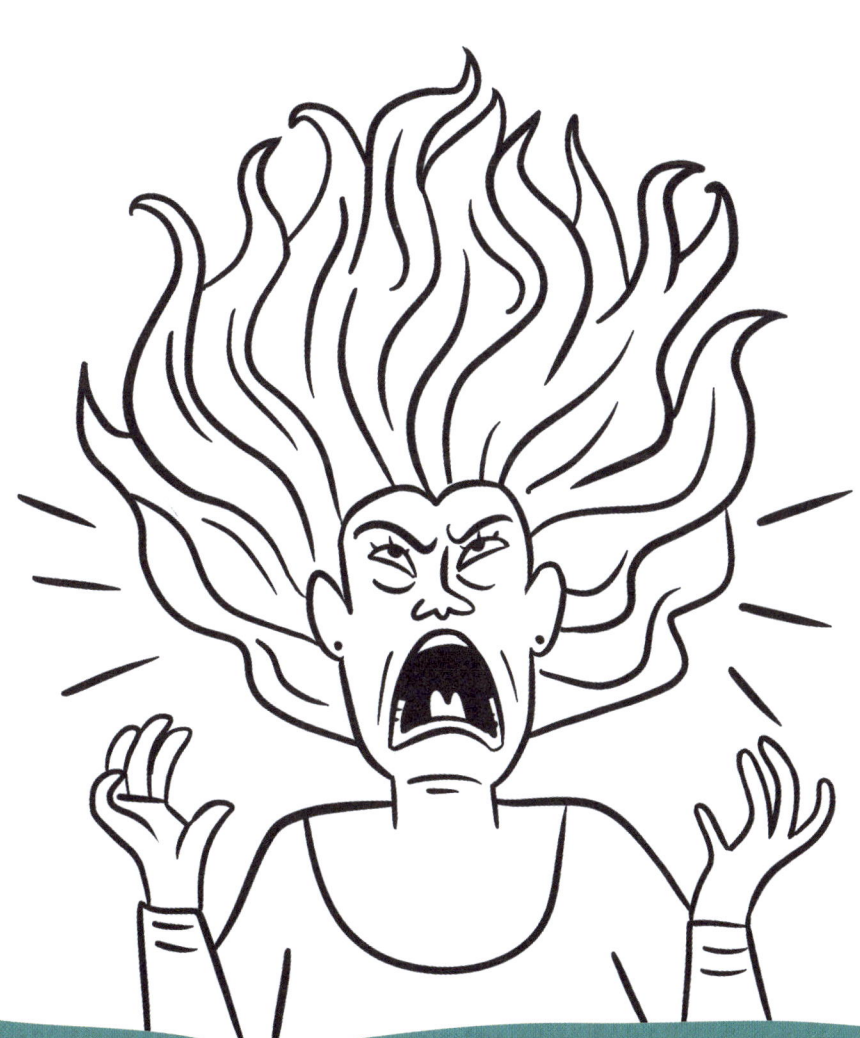

SHAKESPEAREAN MIC DROPS: PART II

The Bard is back with more witty repartee for all of us menopausal matrons. Prepare your next quip for when someone dares ask you how you're feeling.

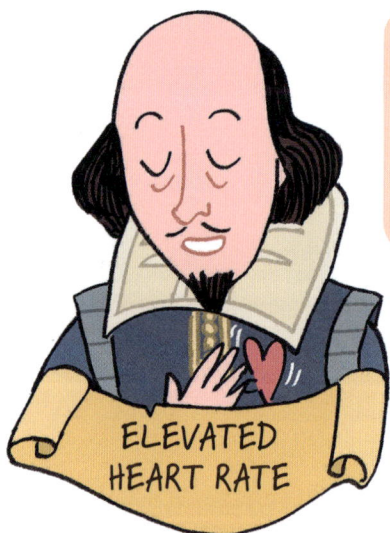

ELEVATED HEART RATE

> I cannot weep; for all my body's moisture
> Scarce serves to quench my furnace-burning heart
> —*Henry VI*

> Too much of water hast thou, poor Ophelia.
> —*Hamlet*

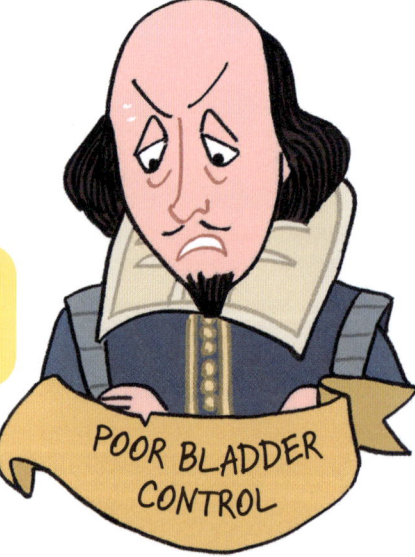

POOR BLADDER CONTROL

> I am sick and sullen.
> —*Antony and Cleopatra*

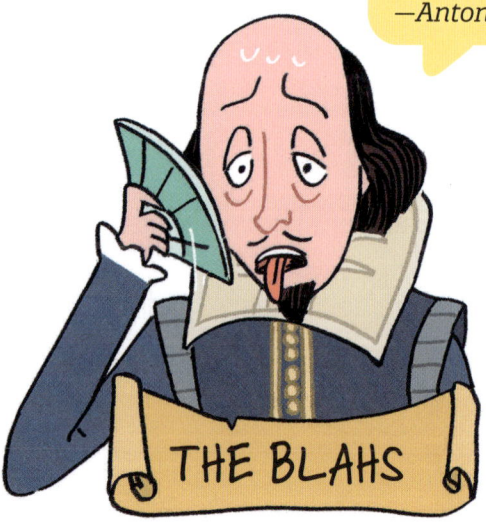

THE BLAHS

> This is enough to be the decay of lust and late-walking through the realm.
> —*The Merry Wives of Windsor*

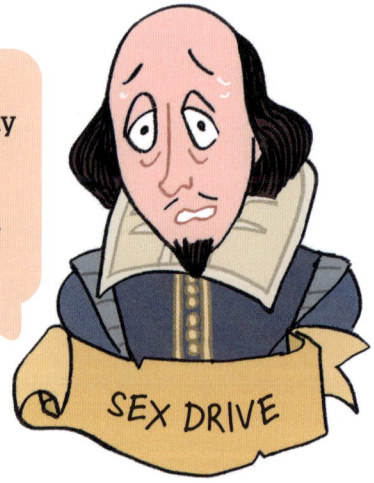

SEX DRIVE

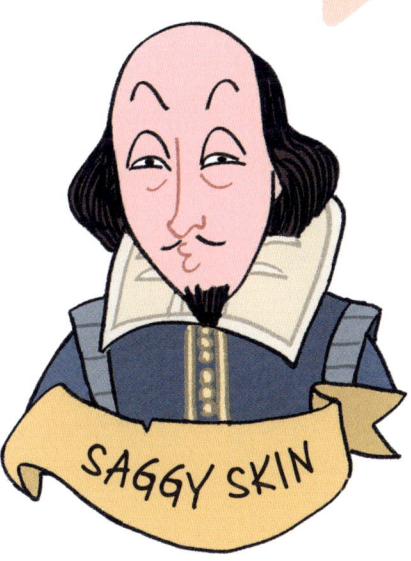

Why, my skin hangs about me like an old lady's loose gown.
—*Henry IV*

SAGGY SKIN

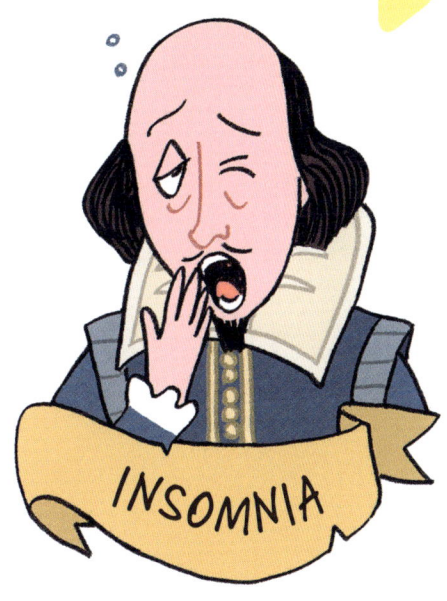

Last night she slept not, nor to-night she shall not.
—*The Taming of the Shrew*

INSOMNIA

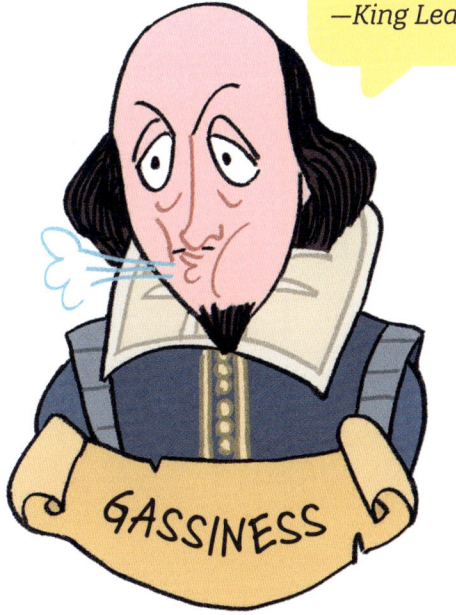

Blow, winds, and crack your cheeks! Rage, blow!
—*King Lear*

GASSINESS

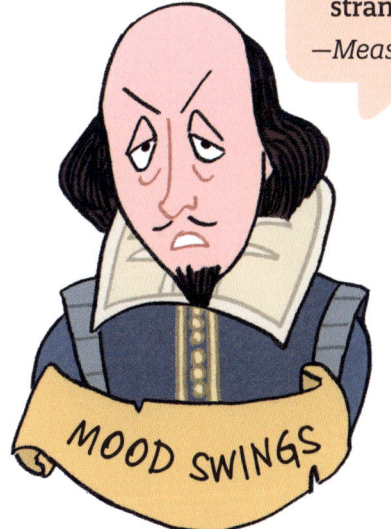

And she will speak most bitterly and strange.
—*Measure for Measure*

MOOD SWINGS

CAN THIS BE NORMAL?

Compare what you're going through with others who have been surveyed. First, answer each question for yourself, then guess the percentage of people who agree with your answer. Regardless of the results, your journey is your own, but it certainly helps to know you're not alone.

1. I didn't know what the difference between perimenopause and menopause was before I started experiencing symptoms myself.

   YES   NO

   Survey says: _____%

2. I think all people experience the same symptoms.

   YES   NO

   Survey says: _____%

3. I get hot flashes.

   YES   NO

   Survey says: _____%

4. I have found my libido dropping since starting perimenopause.

   YES   NO

   Survey says: _____%

5. Hot flashes impact me the most of all peri/menopause symptoms.

   YES   NO

   Survey says: _____%

6. Brain fog impacts me the most of all peri/menopause symptoms.

   YES   NO

   Survey says: _____%

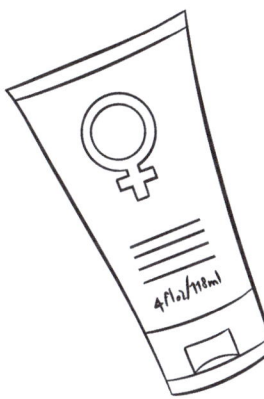

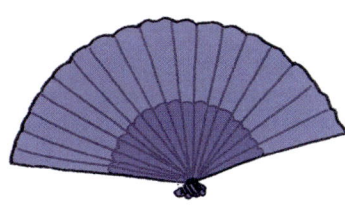

7. Weight gain has the biggest impact on me out of all peri/menopause symptoms.

   YES   NO

   Survey says: _____%

8. Difficulty with sleep impacts me the most of all peri/menopause symptoms.

   YES   NO

   Survey says: _____%

9. I am treating my peri/menopause symptoms.

   YES   NO

   Survey says: _____%

10. I was not prepared for how disruptive menopausal symptoms would be.

    YES   NO

    Survey says: _____%

Answers on page 95.

PUBERTY VS. PERIMENOPAUSE ME

There are many similarities between the phase of life where our reproductive system kicks into gear and the one where it decides to quit. Think back to your days of puberty for the first half, and now for the second. What changes did you start noticing in your body? What filled your thoughts? What did you love? What were you nervous about? How about now? Fill them in!

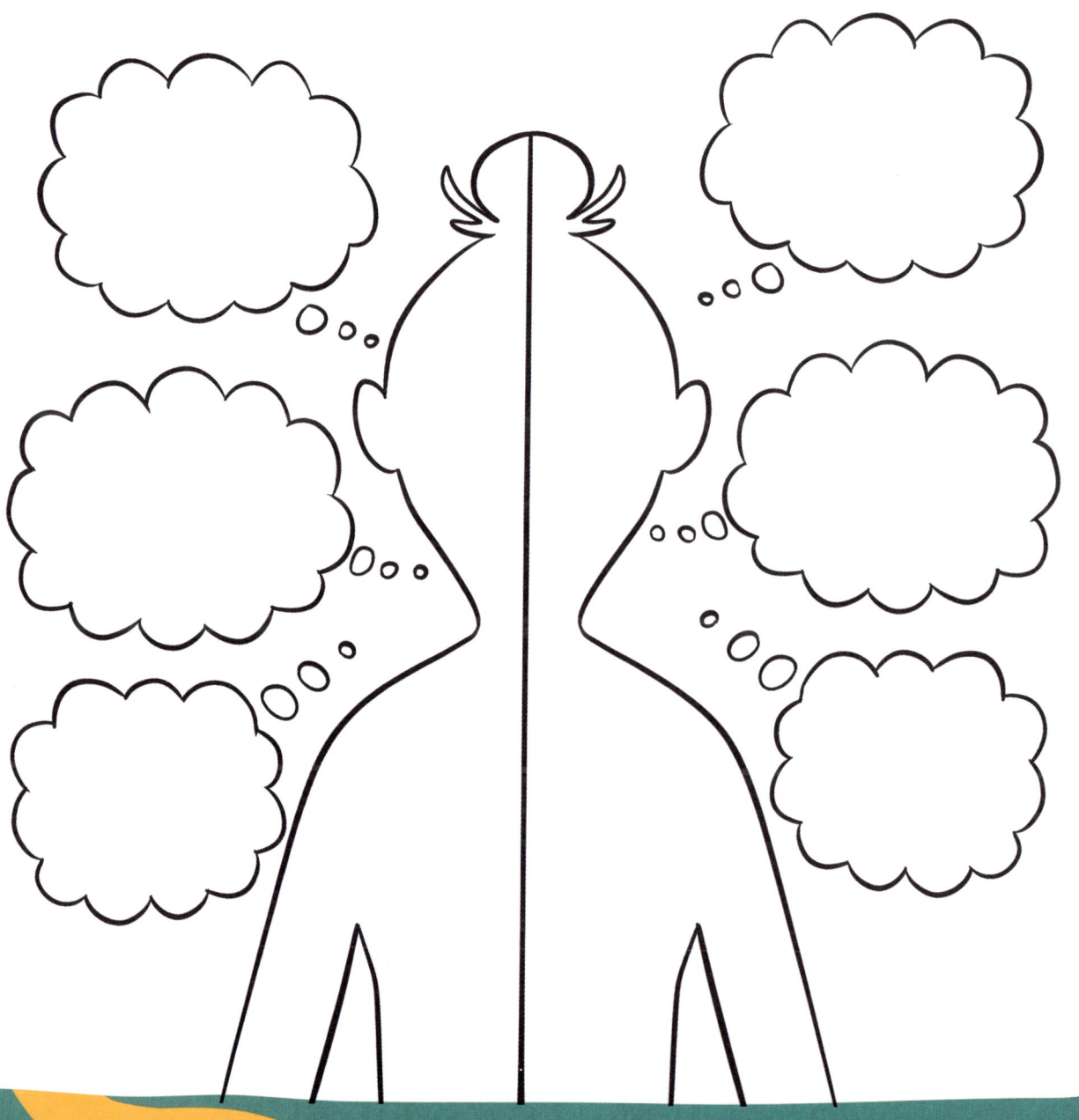

THINGS I WON'T NEED AFTER MENOPAUSE

Oh, happy day, when I can throw these things away! Take a close look at these items and then see if you can answer the questions on the next page.

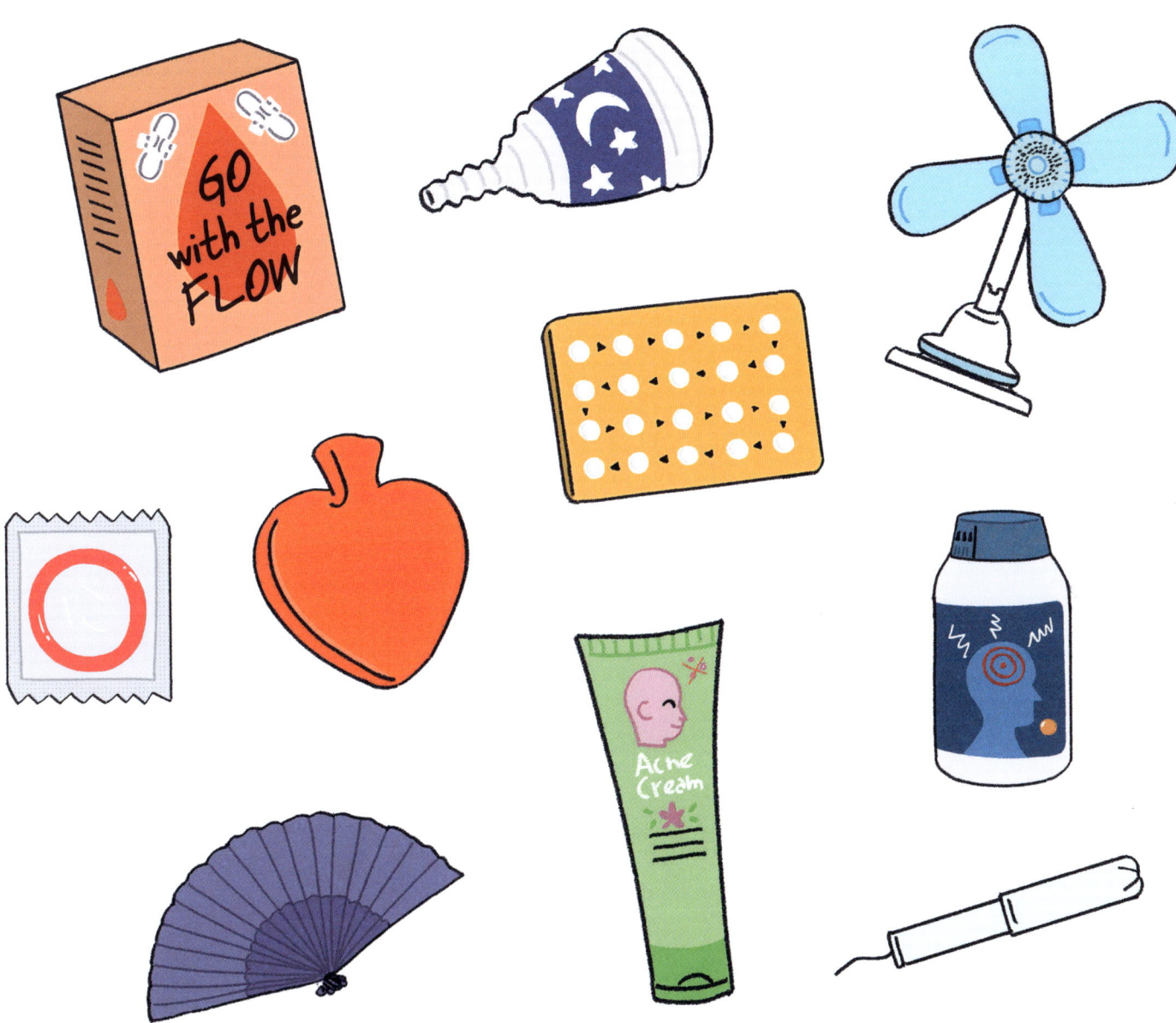

Think about the picture you studied on the previous page, and answer as many of these questions as you can!

List all ten of the things shown that you won't need after menopause (1 point each)

_____   _____

_____   _____

_____   _____

_____   _____

_____   _____

What was the brand name on the sanitary pad? (1 point) _____

How many pills were in the birth control pack? (1 point) _____

How many blades were on the electric fan? (1 point) _____

What was inscribed on the menstrual cup? (1 point) _____

What shape was the hot water bottle? (1 point) _____

TOTAL: _____

Answers on page 95.

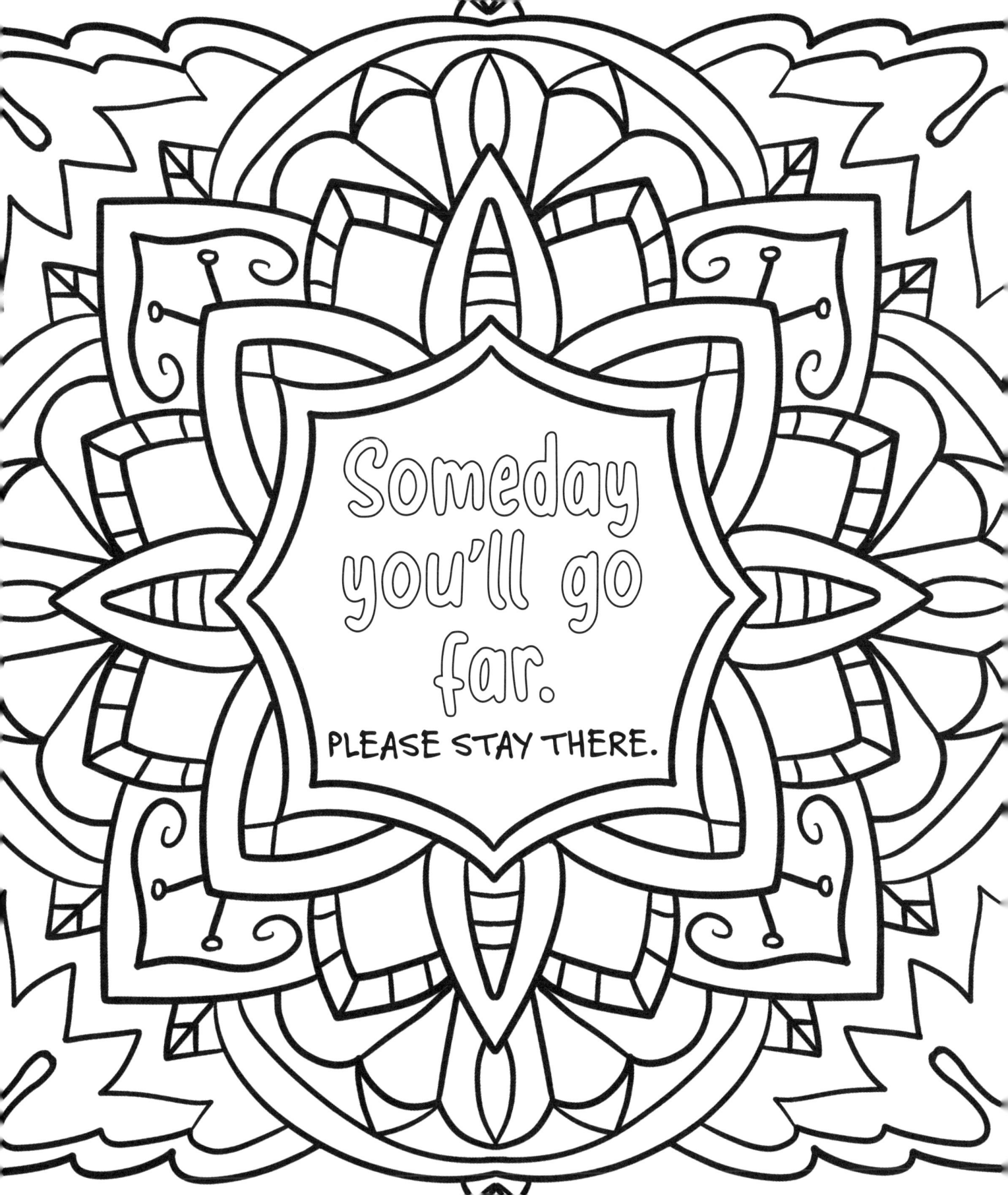

THREE TIPS TO BANISH INVISIBILITY

It's no fun vying for service, being cut in line, or not being taken seriously. Here are three ways to say "HELLO, I'm here!" without actually shouting it.

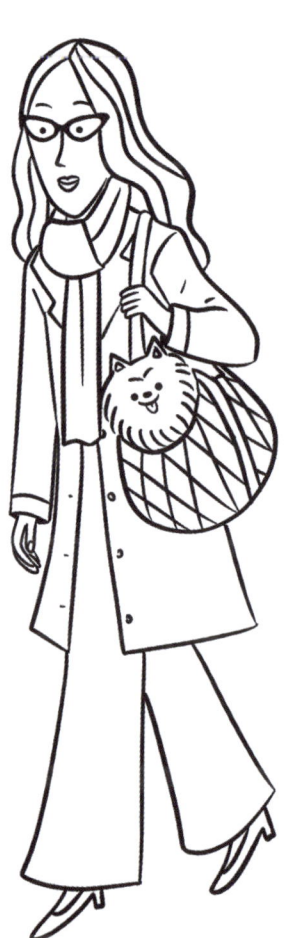

WEAR NEON EVERYTHING.

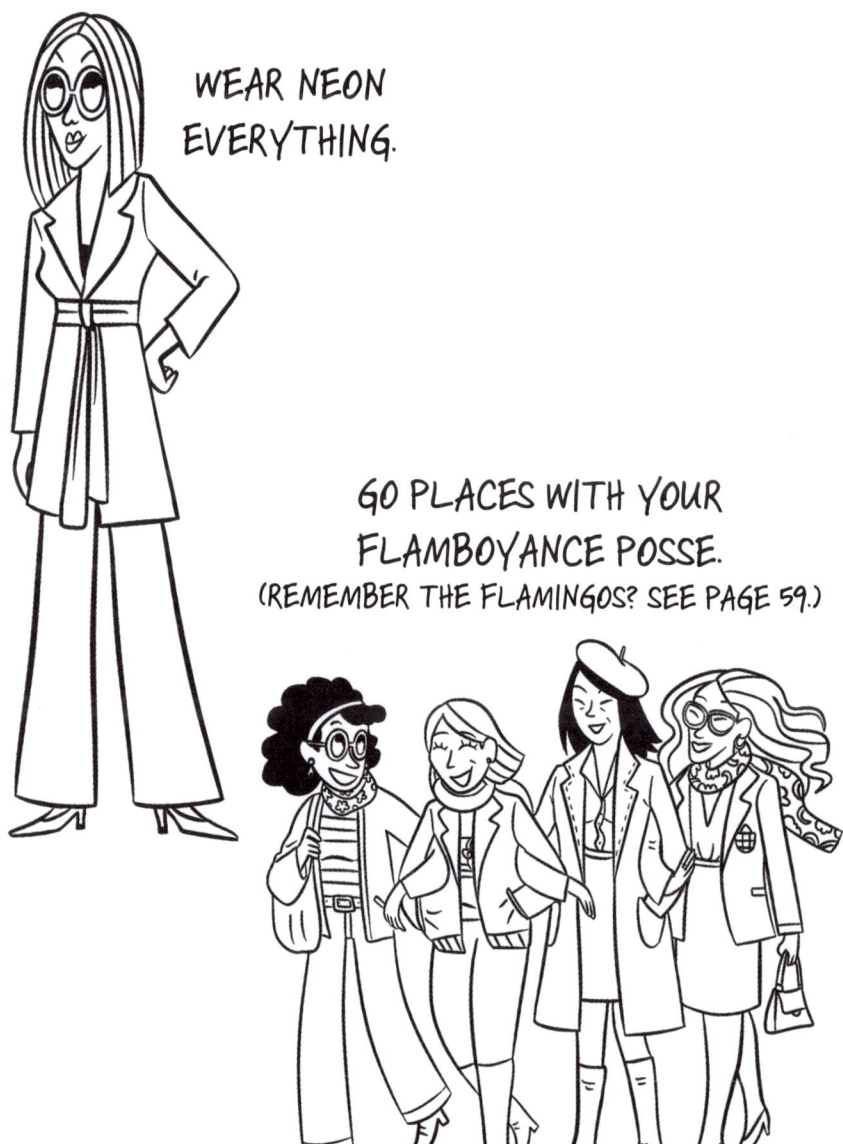

GO PLACES WITH YOUR FLAMBOYANCE POSSE.
(REMEMBER THE FLAMINGOS? SEE PAGE 59.)

GET A POMERANIAN AND CARRY IT EVERYWHERE (IMPOSSIBLE TO IGNORE THE CUTENESS!).

AND THREE TIPS TO EMBRACE INVISIBILITY

Sometimes flying under the radar can be a good thing. Use this new superpower to . . .

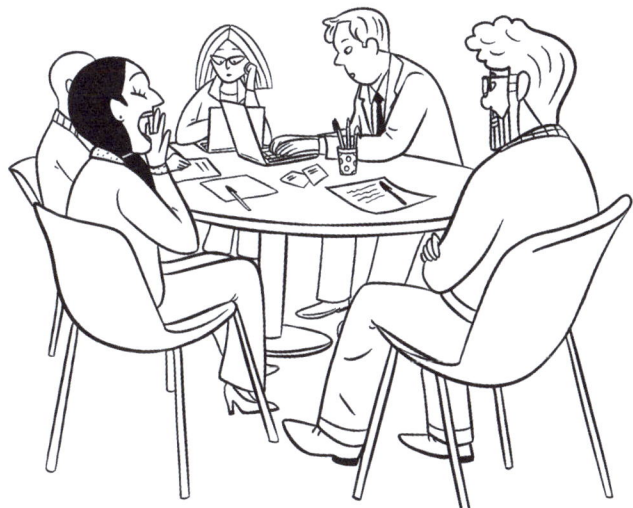

AVOID BORING WORK MEETINGS

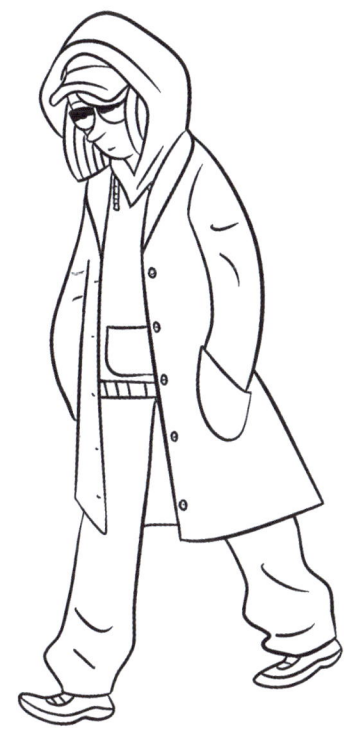

LEAVE THE HOUSE AS-IS

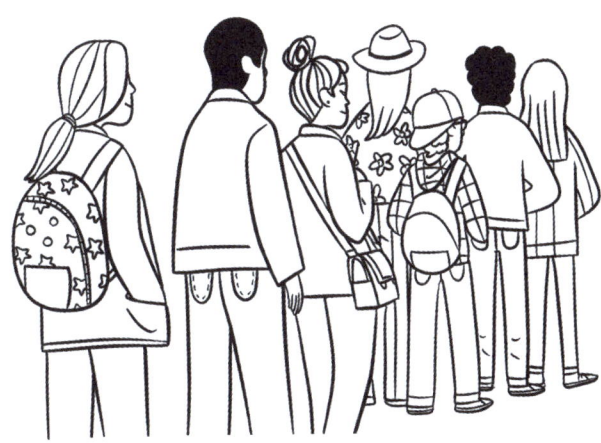

CUT THE LINE

PERI-PERSONALITY

Glass half-empty or half-full? It's all in the attitude! Are you a Doomsday Diva or do you take it all in stride? Complete the quiz to find out . . .

1. **Your girlfriend has been caught out by her period while out with you. What do you do?**

   a. Take off one of your socks to give her, and explain that sometimes, we just have to make do with what we've got.

   b. Tell her to deal with it and be grateful she still gets periods. Soon, they'll all be gone, along with her youth and vigor. Then order yourself the strongest drink on the menu and cry into it.

   c. Shriek with delight, "Your period caught you off guard? It's irregular? Honey, that means you're in PERIMENOPAUSE! Welcome to the club! No, I don't have any spares, sorry."

   d. Tell her about all your surprise periods, complete with the cramps, bloat, clotting, mood swings, and embarrassing moments they each brought.

   e. Give her a pad or tampon you have in your bag, saying, "I never know when mine will hit, so I always have something on hand. You're welcome."

2. **You put on your favorite pair of pants, but they don't fit anymore. What do you do?**

   a. Laugh and take an unflattering selfie with you spilling out of them to share with your bestie. "Yep—death to another wardrobe staple. Do you want them?"

   b. Slump to the floor and caress the pants, remembering all the happy memories you had while wearing them. Then put them back with your other clothes, because you're bound to fit into them again soon.

   c. Smile, grit your teeth, draw a deep breath, suck in your gut, and GET THEM ON! It might take twenty minutes. You might hear some ripping and popping, but you will not give up. These are your pants and nothing will stand in your way of wearing them! Once on, you can hardly breathe or move, but you congratulate yourself for not giving up before staggering for a few steps, then fainting.

   d. Your howl of despair echoes across mountaintops around the country. Expect to spend the next day sitting in your underpants, eating chocolate ice cream while watching trash on TV and feeling sorry for yourself.

   e. You sigh, then put on your trusty track pants and donate the ill-fitting pants to a secondhand store.

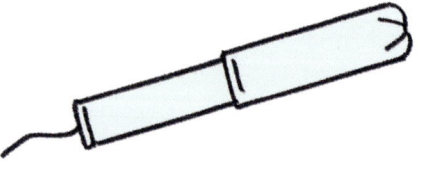

3. **A young, gorgeous thing has been given the promotion at work that everyone knows you deserve. What do you do?**

a. Walk around the workplace, making faces at people and purposely bumping into them. "Oh, my bad. Sorry, I thought I was invisible!"

b. Wear your most revealing clothes to work the next day and bitch to anyone in your way that you've still got what it takes to turn heads. Get grumpy when colleagues turn their backs on you.

c. Print out sheets of flowery affirmations and pin them all over your workspace, and virtually all over your social media. Repeat them under your breath as a mantra, especially when you see that vixen walking past, doing what should be your job.

d. Use your young colleague's photo as a dartboard, give her the evil eye whenever you see her at work, feel sorely tempted to spit in her coffee when her back is turned, then realize it's not so much her, but society. So you have a rant on social media and to anyone who will listen, then console yourself by remembering her boobs will drop one day, too. Unless they're plastic, which they probably are, the tart.

e. You feel punched in the guts. You know it's not fair and you say so in an email to your boss and HR. Then you wipe your eyes and start looking for another job.

4. **You're in a foul mood, and there's no reason why. What do you do?**

a. Make a disclaimer badge to wear, saying you take no responsibility for how your mood swing is making you act. Then have at it—people have been warned, after all.

b. Watch a nostalgic movie from your youth and cry at each scene that reminds you of less turbulent times—conveniently forgetting how periods in your twenties made you a moody thing, too!

c. Fake it till you make it. Plaster on that toothy smile! Open up those eyes! Rebuke those negative thoughts and glide into the day, showering rainbows of positivity and "I've got this" on anyone you meet. Except for that stupid ***** who just looked at you funny. No—breathe . . . breathe . . . deny the feelings and SMILE!

d. Watch out, world. Here comes Hurricane *(insert your name here)*.

e. Snap at a loved one, then apologize and explain that you can't snap out of a rotten mood—it's not their fault at all, but it's best that they give you a bit of space.

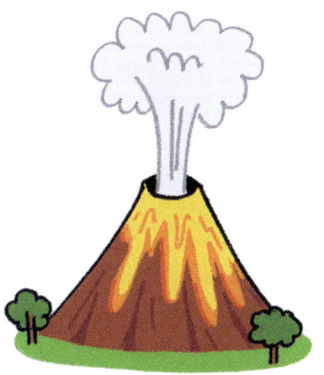

5. You're about to reach the front of a long checkout line, and you suddenly feel a desperate need to pee. What do you do?

a. Groan loudly, then waddle dramatically (and desperately) to the store toilet, clenching your bladder and teeth while squeaking, "Emergency, coming through, excuse me" the whole time. Reach the door, throw it open, and slam it shut behind you—JUST. IN. TIME.

b. Close your eyes and wish yourself back to happier days when you had more bladder control. When that doesn't work, duck out of line and run to the bathroom.

c. Smile serenely at others in the line, while executing a few Kegel exercises discreetly. When that fails and your eyes start watering, suck in a breath between your teeth and smile some more. Finally, when the dam is about to break, sweetly excuse yourself for just a moment, and disguise your desperate need to get to the bathroom by walking with quick, pinched steps, thighs tightly squeezed together, beaming like a newly crowned royal to all you pass on the way.

d. Swear out loud and run to the bathroom, cursing and shoving those in front of you all the way. This is an emergency—MOVE!

e. Invite the person behind you to move ahead of you and watch your cart, then hurry to the restroom. Stop to get some incontinence pads and new underwear on the way to the checkout.

6. You meet a young mother with her baby. What do you do?

a. Commiserate with her about sleepless nights, tender breasts, a changed shape, and feelings of exhaustion all the time. Tell her she has this to look forward to at your age too, minus the baby.

b. Tell her your stories of pregnancy and birth, child-rearing, schools, slumber parties, first dates, family holidays, sending them off to college. Stop for breath, then notice that she's not standing next to you anymore.

c. Gently caress her abdomen and praise her for reaching the zenith of womanhood. Wax lyrical about her feminine power—birthing, nurturing, protecting, and providing. Now place her hand on your tummy and pause, inviting her to listen to the universe singing of the circle of life—not the *Lion King* song, but the rhythm of growth and love and Zen and all things floaty. Sigh, gaze into the distance, and softly chant a requiem for your retiring womb, not noticing how this poor woman would rather be anywhere else than right here with you.

d. Tell her that life is all downhill from here. Think your body feels bad now? Just wait.

e. Coo at the baby and ask the mother how she's doing. Smile and empathize. Inside, you feel hurt at your loss of motherhood with menopause, but you enjoy this new life and seeing this young mother regardless.

7. You're spending the day with family for a holiday and wake up to giggles, realizing you had dropped off to sleep on the couch in front of everyone. What do you do?

a. Ask how loudly you were snoring.

b. Remind all those older than you that they have done the same thing before, and tell everyone stories of how you caught Uncle Joe or Grandma having a sneaky snooze in front of the family. Sigh to yourself as you think of how you used to be the life of the party not that long ago, and now you can hardly keep your eyes open, or others interested in your reminiscences.

c. Tell everyone you were just meditating. That was deep breathing you were doing. Too bad they can't connect with their deeper self the way you can. You would do a downward-facing dog pose to punctuate your point, but you're nervous that you might fart, so leave it at that.

d. Yell at everyone to shut up. When they're suffering the way you are, they'll be grateful for any sleep they can get. Roll over and turn your back to them, then groan that they're all keeping you awake and your back hurts on this uncomfortable couch, and demand that someone rub it, then your feet.

e. Wipe the drool from your chin, grin shyly, then excuse yourself and go off to a room for a quiet nap.

8. You're on a video call with colleagues and notice how you look more aged. What do you do?

a. Put on a silly filter and apologize: "Gee, I'm sorry. I don't know how to take this off!"

b. Lose track of all that is said in the meeting because you're far too busy looking at all the smooth skin, taut eyelids, and stretch-free necks of your colleagues, remembering how you used to look that way too, not that long ago. Make a mental note to research Botox® or even look up a plastic surgeon to see what options you have.

c. Demand a chance to speak. As a senior member of the gathering, impart wisdom to others. It doesn't matter what about. You are wise. Your silver hair and age lines give you the right to be the guru in the room, whether anyone else wants you to or not.

d. Forget that others can see your face too, and spend the meeting looking at your reflection in horror, leaning in close and furrowing your brows to see your wrinkles, then examining your neck wobbles. When a colleague asks what you're doing, close the meeting app immediately in horror at what you've done.

e. Turn off your camera and continue with the meeting.

Which letter did you answer the most? Turn to page 95 to see the menopausal personality others are most likely to see in you.

ANSWER KEY

What Will My Day Look Like?
page 7

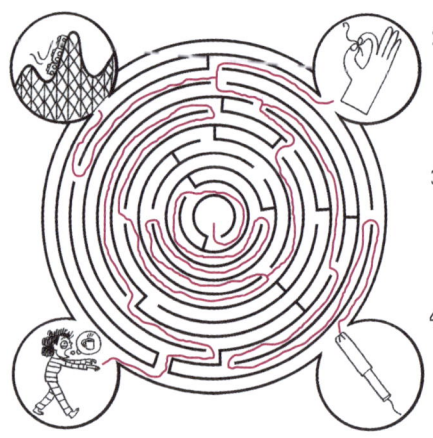

Celebrities—They're Just Like Us
page 8

1. Joan Rivers, 2. Michelle Obama, 3. Emma Thompson, 4. Angelina Jolie, 5. Shania Twain, 6. Viola Davis, 7. Michelle Yeoh, 8. Salma Hayek, 9. Oprah Winfrey, 10. Halle Berry, 11. Drew Barrymore

What Was I Thinking?
page 14

keys	birthdays
map	purse
date	remote
names	laundry
appointments	password
words	faces
medication	pen
anniversary	phone
wallet	glasses
address	trash
car	

Secret Phrase:
Your secrets are safe with me. I'll never remember them anyway!

Menopause Myth Busters
page 18

1. B. The first sign that you're entering perimenopause is a change in your period regularity.

2. B. Smoking can increase your risk of menopause before forty-five years old. Drinking, more pregnancies, and going through puberty early can all lead to a LATER onset of menopause.

3. A. Tight clothes can restrict blood flow and make hot flashes worse! Only loose linen for me, please! Now the wardrobe on the *Golden Girls* makes so much more sense.

4. C. If you've put on a few pounds, you are not alone, sister! On average, women gain 12 to 15 pounds between forty-five and fifty-five, and it tends to accumulate around your middle. It's not you, it's the time of life!

5. C. No bronchitis, but is that a ringing in your ears? Yes, yes it is. Tinnitus is a lesser known symptom of menopause. About 15 percent of women get a painful little warning that a hot flash is coming courtesy of an electric shock. If you're wondering what burning tongue is, about 10 percent of women experience a metallic taste and dry or sore tongue due to pain-sensitive nerves around your taste buds.

6. B. It takes on average four years to go through perimenopause but it can range from a few months to over ten years.

7. C. Technically, all the fun you experience while you're still getting a period—albeit irregularly—is perimenopause. You have to have not gotten a visit from Aunt Flo for a year for it to be classified as menopause.

8. B. The average hot flash lasts 4 minutes, though some hot flashes may only last for a few seconds and others can go for more than 10 minutes.

9. D. Your heart rate can increase by 8 to 16 beats per minute during a hot flash. That racing heart is not your imagination.

10. C. The only other mammals we know of who undergo menopause are short fin pilot whales and false killer whales. This means they live longer than their reproductive ability. Other mammals are able to have babies till the day they die. No, thanks!

By Any Other Name
page 22

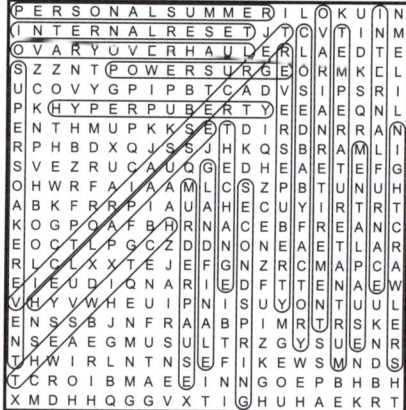

Stop the Leaks Maze!
page 23

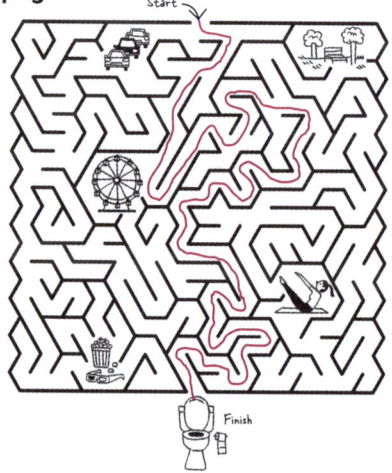

Menopause Marquee
page 25

There is no more creative force in the world than the menopausal woman with zest.

—Margaret Mead

Tricky Terminology
page 26

1. B. Oogenesis is the production of egg cells, which ends with menopause.

2. C. Climacteric is the time of life when fertility is at a decline, a synonym for menopause.

3. A. Psychoneuroendocrinology is a field of research that studies how hormones can impact mental illness.

4. B. Osteopenia is the loss of bone mineral density, which often occurs during menopause.

5. A. Progesterone is the hormone that prepares the lining of the uterus for an egg to grow. When this is lowered, it can result in hot flashes, weight gain, mood fluctuations, irregular periods, trouble sleeping, headaches, and more.

6. D. Premature ovarian insufficiency, or POI, is a loss of ovarian function in those younger than forty.

7. B. Hormone replacement therapy, or HRT, is used to alleviate estrogen deficiency symptoms.

8. C. Telogen effluvium is hair loss due to an imbalanced hair growth cycle. In perimenopause, this can be due to dropping estrogen levels.

Hormonal Powder Keg
page 32

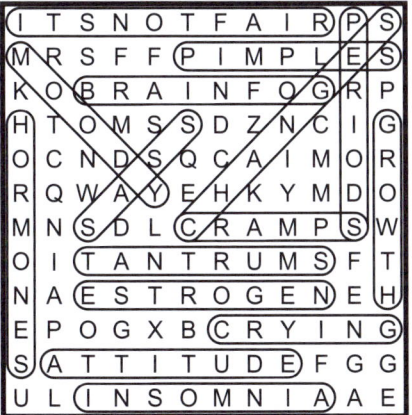

Where Did I Put My Keys?
page 33

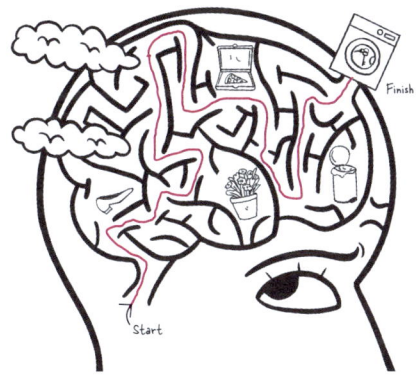

Natural Ways to Reduce Symptoms
page 42

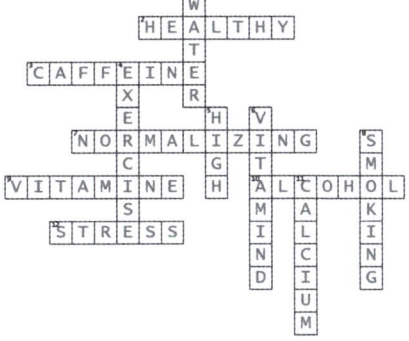

House Partay!
page 44

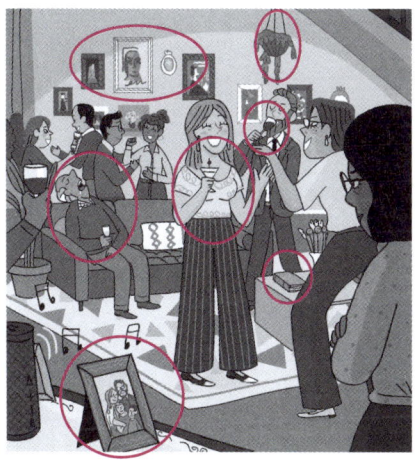

I Am Amazing!
page 50

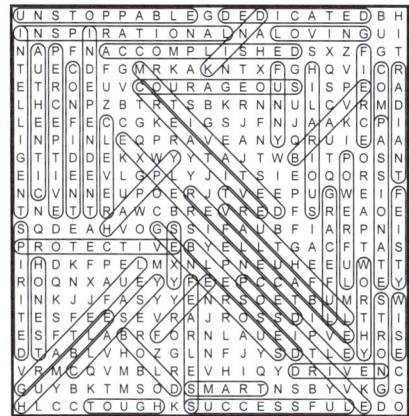

Symptom Scramble
page 54

Halitosis
Fatigue
Insomnia
Constipation
Nausea
Itchiness
Tinnitus
Osteoporosis
Headaches
Anxiety

A Hot Flash-back Through History
page 60

1. C. 1821 by French physician Charles-Pierre-Louis de Gardanne

2.

Month of Stopping	Greek
Second Spring	Chinese
Years of Renewing Energy	Japanese
The Hopeless Age	Arabic

3. D. 1940s—this was turned into what became a very popular drug in the United States, Premarin®, which is still used today.

4. C. Soy contains isoflavones, which mimic estrogen, so when estrogen lowers during menopause, its effects are less noticeable.

5. A. Cow ovaries were turned into Ovariin in the 1890s, and testicular extract was also advocated as a treatment.

6. C. Black or Hispanic

7. D. It's horrifying, I know!

8. A, though the other answers were true for other cultures. B was true in in Cambodian history; C was true as published by seventeenth-century physician Nicolaas Fonteyn in his book, *The Womans Doctour*; D was published in E. J. Tilt's *The Change of Life in Health and Disease* (1857).

9. C. How poetic . . .

10. B. He also believed they could turn wine to vinegar, make crops wither, and dim mirrors!

Forty Symptoms for the Over-Forty Crowd
page 62

Menopause Watching
page 65

1. 3
2. 2
3. Flowers
4. Hang out in the freezer section
5. Checkout operator
6. Ketchup
7. Candy
8. Hot flashes, fatigue, irritability, and so many more!

Tales of Transformation
page 68

A	**Meno-Mummy:** You hardly function, except to wander from your bed or the couch to the toilet, multiple times. Discourse toward you will be answered with noncommittal grunts as you shuffle and trip over yourself to get to your favorite destination—anywhere that's quiet where you can be horizontal, undisturbed, with eyes closed.
B	**Inferni, the Hellgal:** You once were hot in quite a different way. Now, you sizzle and roast with your internal inferno, scorching anyone who crosses you unawares or dares suggest it's all in your head. Seldom seen without your fan.
C	**The Blob:** Similar to the Marshmallow Man from *Ghostbusters*, nobody dare bust you, or your bust might bust them back! A wobbly mass of destruction, you shun societal expectations and embrace the body time has gifted you, dry skin, varicose veins, chin hairs, and all.
D	**The Dried Bride of Frankenstein:** You feel like a botched jumble, put together haphazardly. Nothing works right anymore. You creak and everything hurts. Frequently found at the medicine or wine cabinet, or roaming the neighborhood, groaning for sympathy and asking for a back rub.
E	**Creature of the Fog:** You exist in a perpetual mist, aimlessly stumbling and constantly wondering what you were meant to be doing. In the rare moments when the fog clears, you set off with purpose, only for the fog to envelop you once again, sending you haplessly in random directions.
F	**PeriDactyl:** You screech, you swoop, and anyone daring to mess with you is likely to be severely pecked. At times graceful and elegant, up close, you're mostly terrifying, especially to those you've randomly selected to be prey. (And woe to all who say you're from the time of the dinosaurs!)

Can This Be Normal?
page 80

1. 55% know the difference between perimenopause and menopause before experiencing it themselves.

2. About 33% of menopausal people believe everyone's experiences are the same. They're not. There are thirty-four recognized symptoms, and while some might get them all, others get none. (Lucky buggers!!)

3. Over 80% of those in peri/menopause get hot flashes.

4. 43% have found their libido dropping since starting perimenopause.

5. Hot flashes are the symptom with the biggest impact on 13% of those in perimenopause and 16% in menopause.

6. Brain fog is the symptom with the biggest impact on 11% of those in perimenopause and 10% in menopause.

7. Weight gain is the symptom with the biggest impact on 15% of those in peri/menopause.

8. Sleep difficulty is the symptom with the biggest impact on 14% of those in peri/menopause.

9. 27% of peri/menopausal people are not treating their symptoms.

10. 63% of peri/menopausal people didn't feel prepared for how disruptive menopausal symptoms would be.

Things I Won't Need After Menopause
page 83

Sanitary pad, tampon, menstrual cup, birth control, condom, headache tablets, hot water bottle, electric fan, hand fan, acne cream

Go with the Flow

20

4

Moon and stars

Heart

How did you do out of 15 points?

0–5: Oh dear. You might need to keep these things for a while longer yet, as it seems that you're smack bang still in the middle of all the symptoms. But don't worry, the brain fog will clear. It is a temporary hormonal barb of menopause, not dementia. You'll be all right—in time.

6–10: Pretty good work there! Seems like there's still some menopausal memory-mulch for you, but you're working through it. The light at the end of the tunnel is coming—really!

11–15: You are the ringmaster with a well-trained brain! Are you still needing anything on this list, or are you waltzing happily out of menopause already? Lucky you, if so. At any rate, your memory seems good for now. Yay!

Peri-Personality
page 88

A	**The Humorist:** It's here, and it's not all fun, but you do what you have to do to keep a smile on your face and a sense of sanity in it all. Some days, that's easier than others!
B	**The Time Warper:** Your mind and heart are in the past, back when you were young, firm, and fertile. Reality now is less pleasant, so any reminder of it is bound to bring tension.
C	**The Over-Optimist:** You've read every self-help and positive mindset book relating to menopause there is, you shut out any negative thought or mention of symptoms, and you are ready to OWN IT! (Frankly, this book would be torture for you. I'm surprised you've gotten this far.)
D	**The Doomsday Diva:** Your. World. Is. Ending! And no, you won't be quiet about your dry skin or latest symptom.
E	**The Plodder:** You don't make a fuss, or want to be the center of attention, but damn, these symptoms are no fun.

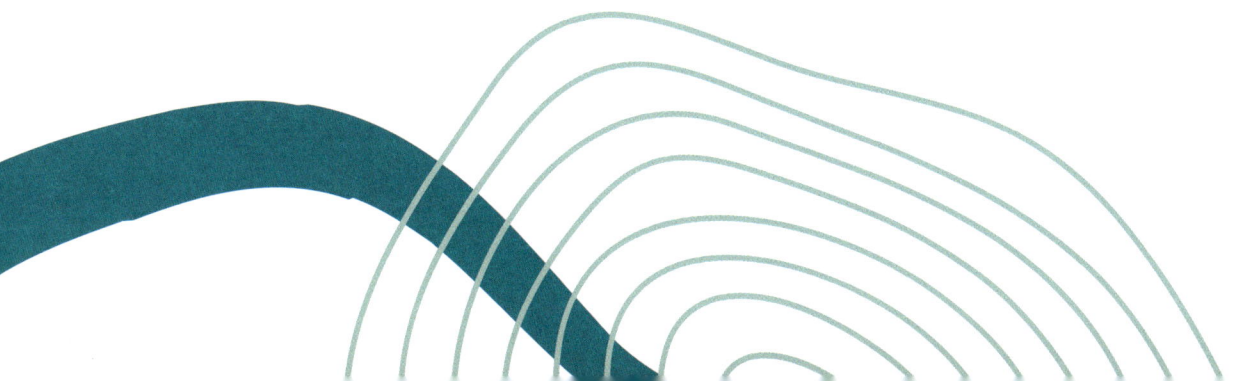

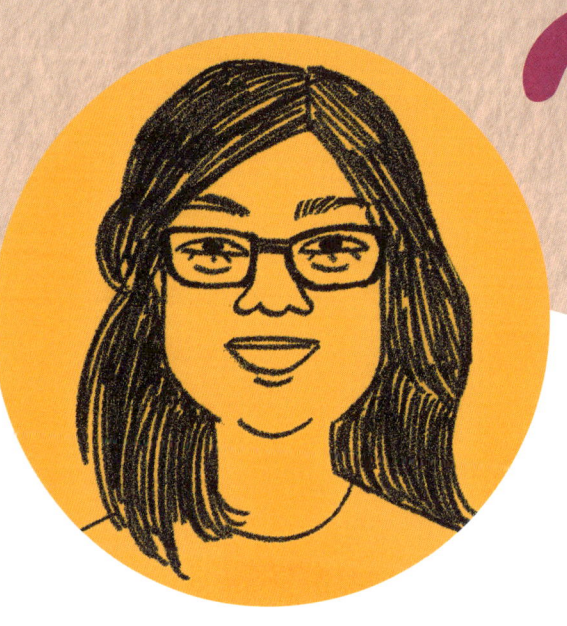

ABOUT THE AUTHOR

SHIRLEY ȘERBAN is a middle-aged New Zealander in perimenopause, a writer, and comedy songwriter. She has a love of laughing with others at the joys of aging, housework, dealing with other people, and all the challenges life throws our way. In May 2021, Shirley created a parody song on YouTube, called "Menopause Rhapsody," based on the Queen classic, which has since reached over eight million views, garnered a lot of media attention, and made Shirley the unofficial face of menopause comedy. Find out more on her website, www.shirleycan.com and on her YouTube channel @ShirleySerban.